HOW I ROLL

*life, love, & work
after a spinal
cord injury*

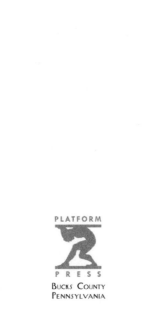

PLATFORM

PRESS

BUCKS COUNTY
PENNSYLVANIA

HOW I ROLL

life, love, & work after a spinal cord injury

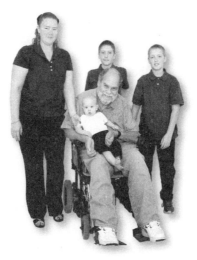

J. BRYANT NEVILLE, JR.
with
Raquel B. Pidal

Published in the United States by Platform Press, an imprint of
Winans Kuenstler Publishing, LLC, Doylestown, Pennsylvania
www.WKPublishing.com
Inquire about discounts for bulk orders.

Visit HowIRollBook.com for current information about author
appearances, news, and links to resources.

Visit SpinalCord.org for information and resources for people
affected by spinal cord injury, multiple sclerosis, polio,
amyotrophic lateral sclerosis, and spina bifida, and those who
love and help them.

Cover photos: © Heather Perry

Printed in the United States of America

Dedicated to the many people who have helped me learn that the powers of grace and love make all things possible.

acknowledgments

There are so many parts involved in bringing a story to life in a way that will both interest and entice the reader—parts I never knew existed until embarking on this project in July of 2010. There are some very important people I wish to thank, without whom I could not deliver what I pray is a message of hope for those now facing challenges.

Firstly, I wish to thank my family for all the help and support over the past thirty years and for your encouragement and belief in everything I've ever wanted to do—including this book. Without my mom and dad, my wife and three boys, my extended family, my true friends, and my great community, there would be no story worth telling. I am where I am today because of each of you, and I will never be able to amply thank you.

Secondly, I want to express my sincerest thanks to Paul Tobin, President of the United Spinal Association, and Eric Larson, former President of the National Spinal Cord Injury Association, which recently merged with United Spinal and now represents its outreach arm under his continued leadership. Together, these two gentlemen have demonstrated a tremendous belief in a story they feel worthy of telling as an inspirational and motivational tool for those facing life with a spinal cord injury.

Evidencing their support is a commitment to purchase the initial 5,000 copies for the newly injured and as a resource for individual member chapters. I could not have afforded the publishing cost on my own nor could I have accessed a distribution network specifically targeting the audience I feel may be most helped by the book. As we move forward with sales to the general public, 40% of the net revenues will go toward supporting the national mission of United Spinal, and 10% of the net revenues will go toward the support of the Virginia state chapter's mission.

Thirdly, none of this would have begun had it not been for the eager response by Foster Winans, President and Chief Creative Officer of Winans Kuenstler Publishing, to a short paragraph pitching my story. We talked, and after he'd listened to my concepts, he quickly acknowledged a desire to help me with the project, worked out an affordable budget, and assigned Raquel Pidal to help me bring my words to life. I could not have penned my humble tale without the help and support of these two dedicated people, and I have thoroughly enjoyed working with them both.

I have no doubt that there are some people I have overlooked so please forgive me if you are one of them. To those mentioned above as well as anyone I may have forgotten, take comfort in the knowledge that your involvement in my life has inspired me to try and help others.

contents

author's note xi

spinal cord injury facts xiv

message from NSCIA xv

foreword: dr. dan gottlieb xvii

prologue: impact................................... xxiii

chapter 1: farm boy................................. 27

chapter 2: a girlfriend and a car.......... 36

chapter 3: losing control...................... 46

chapter 4: lightning strikes................. 51

chapter 5: a plate of french fries 64

chapter 6: tough love............................ 82

chapter 7: more than a hatrack 95

chapter 8: college days........................ 109

chapter 9: banking on the future........ 124

chapter 10: filling the void 143

chapter 11: a dream fulfilled 165

epilogue: 187

resources.. 189

author's note

Thirty years ago, my life was turned upside down when an auto accident left me a quadriplegic, paralyzed from the neck down, at age 17.

In the blink of an eye, my lifelong dreams of a family of my own and a career to support them seemed dashed. I was confused, frightened, angry—questioning my faith and existence. I was blessed to have the unending love and support of the greatest parents in the world, a huge extended family, a host of friends, and an amazing community. Because of these great people, I was able to find strength to accept my new way of life and regain the faith to believe that I could still achieve my goals. The road was rough, and tears were shed along the way, but the dreams I'd once thought out of my reach have become my reality.

When I was first injured, my Aunt Betty gave me a wall hanging she had cross-stitched of the poem on the next page. I hung it where I could read it daily, and it inspired me to keep going, even when I questioned whether it was worthwhile.

It is my humble hope that sharing my journey will help those who are just beginning theirs to believe in life's endless possibilities, no matter what challenges they may face. I hope my words capture the essence of the poem my aunt gave me: that you will discover purpose in what may seem like a meaningless existence, if you only think you can.

—J. Bryant Neville, Jr.
DeWitt, Virginia

thinking

If you think you are beaten, you are,
If you think you dare not, you don't.
If you like to win, but you think you can't,
It is almost certain you won't.

If you think you'll lose, you're lost,
For out in the world we find,
Success begins with a fellow's will.
It's all in the state of mind.

If you think you are outclassed, you are,
You've got to think high to rise,
You've got to be sure of yourself before
You can ever win a prize.

Life's battles don't always go
To the stronger or faster man.
But soon or late the man who wins,
Is the man who thinks he can.

—Walter D. Wintle
circa 1905

spinal cord injury facts

- There are about **12,000** new cases of spinal cord injury each year—an average of **33 new injuries a day**.
- About **265,000** Americans have a spinal cord injury.
- **80%** are male.
- Spinal cord injuries are most commonly caused by:
  Vehicular accidents: **40%**
  Falls: **28%**
  Violence: **15%**
  Sports: **8%**
  Other: **9%**
- The average age at injury is currently **40 years**.
- Among those with a spinal cord injury, when discharged from the hospital:
  —**55%** have quadriplegia (complete or incomplete)
  —**44%** have paraplegia (complete or incomplete)
  —Less than **1%** experience a complete neurologic recovery when discharged.
- Over **57%** of people with a spinal cord injury are employed at the time of injury. One year after injury, **11%** are employed; 20 years after injury, **35%** are employed.
- The average lifetime health and living costs for a person injured with paraplegia at age 25: **$2.1 million**.
- The average lifetime health and living costs for a person injured with quadriplegia at age 25: **$3.1 to $4.3 million**.

Source: National Spinal Cord Injury Statistical Center, Birmingham, Alabama (https://www.nscisc.uab.edu/)
Visit www.spinalcord.org/resource-center/ for more information.

about our community

Learning to adapt to life with a spinal cord injury or disorder may be the greatest challenge anyone can encounter. Having the right support to smooth the bumps in the road back to independence can make the journey much easier and more rewarding.

National Spinal Cord Injury Association (NSCIA) is the membership program of United Spinal Association. Our mission is to improve the quality of life of all people living with spinal cord injuries and disorders (SCI/D). NSCIA has more than 65 years of experience educating and empowering individuals with SCI/D. We have a national network of local chapters and support groups, connecting people with SCI/D to their peers and fostering an expansive grassroots network that enriches lives.

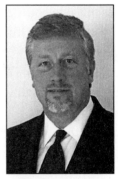

K. Eric Larson

Our membership program is a lifeline for many individuals focused on regaining their independence and improving their quality of life—whether they are leaving rehab after sustaining a spinal cord injury, learning to live with symptoms of a spinal cord disorder, or have spent years coping with disability.

That's why we are so excited to be working with J. Bryant Neville, Jr., on a national initiative built around this book, which chronicles his 30-year journey with a high-level spinal cord injury.

Bryant's willingness to share his story will help us raise awareness of the tremendous possibilities for people with spinal cord injury and disease to achieve a high level of independence, health, and personal fulfillment in their lives—all things Bryant has achieved.

Just as importantly, Bryant is donating a generous portion of the sale of every book to benefit NSCIA and programs like our resource center, Spinal Cord Central, and our New Beginning backpacks, which are filled with essential resources for those newly diagnosed with SCI/D on living a healthy, active lifestyle. These backpacks, given out at hospitals and rehabilitation facilities, help those with SCI/D unlock opportunities to achieve goals that might otherwise be unattainable.

If you know or meet someone living with a spinal cord injury or disorder, please give them a copy of this book and refer them to us.

K. Eric Larson
SVP Membership and Chapter Services
NSCIA, a program of United Spinal Association

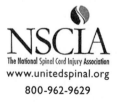

NSCIA
The National Spinal Cord Injury Association
www.unitedspinal.org
800-962-9629

foreword: dr. dan gottlieb

The story you are about to read begins with an experience strikingly similar to my own—an instant in time that completely changed the course of my life. In 1979, I had an established career as a psychologist and was the father of two little girls when a loose wheel from a tractor trailer smashed into the car I was driving, leaving me paralyzed from the chest down—a condition called quadriplegia.

No amount of knowledge or training prepares you for the physical and emotional challenges of developing a new set of life skills. But I did, like Bryant Neville, have a revelatory moment during my initial hospitalization. One night in intensive care, trussed up in a grotesque apparatus to keep my neck stable, feeling suicidal, a nurse came to my bedside and asked if it was true what she'd heard, that I was a psychologist.

"Yes," I answered.

Knowing nothing of my state of mind, she asked, "Does everyone feel suicidal at some point in their life?"

"Well, it's not unusual," I replied. "But if you want to

talk, come back after your shift."

She did come back, pulled up a chair, and we talked into the night. She told me about her life, and I referred her to a therapist. When she left, I closed my eyes and thought, "I can live with this." That woman saved my life because she asked something of me and allowed herself to be vulnerable.

Bryant Neville was only 17 years old but he saved his own life by asking something of himself—he was determined to disprove a doctor's grim prognosis. Thirty years later, in his unflinching look at what quadriplegia has been like for him, he has allowed himself to be vulnerable, revealing intimate details without self-pity.

Some will read this story and think it's a miracle to survive such an experience and to live as he has. The beauty of his story—the beauty of life itself—is that it's really not a miracle. As surely as a flower is drawn to the sun, it is the calling of the human spirit, regardless of circumstances, to seek wholeness, to thrive, to live, and to find meaning.

In spite of my hospital-room revelatory moment, it took me many years to work through the complex emotions I felt and to understand the complex emotions felt by those who loved me, those who cared for me, and even those who knew me only as a man in a wheelchair. Like Bryant, I have had many experiences when people treated me as if I were deaf and mute or, worse, invisible.

It happened often enough that when I took my young children out to eat, we developed a routine that amused us but usually went over the heads of the staff. The host or hostess would ask the girls, "Where would he like to sit?" They would turn to me and ask, "Where would you like to sit?" I would reply, "I want to sit over there." They would then announce, "He wants to sit over there."

Bryant's depiction of discovering his sexual capabilities was inspiring to me and touches on an issue that needs to be talked about more. When I went through my experience three decades ago, the education about sexual activity and spinal cord impairment was poor. The first time I went to bed with my wife, she began to touch me and I started to cry and said, "Don't touch me where I'm dead."

Many years later, I had a chance to talk about sex with my 82-year-old father, who fancied himself quite the ladies man. He'd had prostate surgery and one day when I was driving him home from an errand in my adapted van, he said, "I don't even know why I flirt anymore. I can't have sex."

I pulled over to the side of the road, turned off the engine, and said, "For the first time in my life, we're going to talk about sex." I described for him what it was like for me—the sounds, the senses, the passion and excitement. "It's not as good as it was before the accident, but it's still damn good." He turned bright red, which I enjoyed.

What do people like us need from those around us? We need people who have faith in us more than we need cheerleaders. Whenever I'm in a dark place, I want to be with someone who loves me enough to sit with me and not tell me it's light outside. I don't want to be told I'm thinking the wrong way or should be feeling differently. All of us in this situation have heard that and what it says to us is that not only are our bodies broken, but there's also something wrong with the way we're thinking. The problem is the spinal cord injury, not the person.

We need to acknowledge and deal with guilt, of which there is plenty to go around. My wife said she felt guilty that she was able to walk. I felt terribly guilty that I was compromising the quality of life for her and our children. To this day, I feel some pain inside about what I was unable to do for my kids. The problem is that chronic pain, emotional as well as physical, can cause us to become self-absorbed and make it harder to love others.

The cure for guilt is to love who we love better. If I could have been my therapist, I would have asked myself, What does your wife really want from you? Try to understand her experience. Try not to let your guilt interfere with your compassion for those you love.

Envy and resentment are other emotions I felt. A month or so after my accident, I was in a rehabilitation facility in an urban neighborhood looking out the window and noticed a homeless man sleeping on a steam vent. I felt envy because he could get up and walk away from his condition. That was the depth of my despair. I don't feel envy of anyone anymore. Like Bryant, I feel grateful for my life. I don't have time to complain about today because everything I have could be gone tomorrow.

A spinal cord injury is a broken promise but few people, including those who love us, can give voice to the fact that they feel betrayed. In the early years, I hated my body for betraying me. And then I feared my body. For many years I resented it. I used to say that my body acted like a terrorist but I treated it like a fickle lover.

After awhile I discovered that it was possible to feel gratitude and compassion for my body. When my body, which has worked so hard, is in crisis, it doesn't understand why. When I get a urinary tract infection or I have neuro-pathic pain in my arms, I feel the same sort of tenderness one feels when seeing an infant suffering—my heart opens up with kindness.

More than three decades after being betrayed by a spinal cord injury, I can say honestly that I have attained a quality of life that is superior to most. I suspect Bryant feels the same way, and, like me, I suspect he is grateful for the body he has.

—Dr. Dan Gottlieb

Dan Gottlieb, Ph.D., a psychotherapist for 40 years in the Philadelphia area, is host of Voices in the Family, *a talk show on public radio station WHYY in Philadelphia, and he is heard weekly on NPR's* Morning Edition. *He is the author of several books including the internationally acclaimed* Letters to Sam, *a collection of lessons on life he wrote to his grandson, published in 1996. He also writes for* The Huffington Post. *His show archives and other information can be found at DrDanGottlieb.com.*

prologue: impact

The first thing I noticed was the silence. It was spring in central Virginia—a chilly March night when the peeper frogs should have been singing their chorus of love songs. But I didn't hear them. All I noticed was that the night was still and pitch black as I slumped against the door of my pickup. I had swerved to avoid hitting a deer, and now my truck rested upside down against a tree.

The next thing I noticed was the strong odor of gasoline. I had to get out before it could ignite.

My brain ordered my arms to reach up and pull myself out through the broken window, but nothing happened. My brain told my legs to push me out—nothing happened. Come on, arms! Come on, legs! Nothing. It was as if my mind and my body were no longer connected.

The only thing I could move was my head. I thrashed my neck around a few times thinking I might dislodge whatever was trapping my arms and legs. Still nothing.

I opened my mouth to shout for help, but nothing came out. The air seemed to slowly leak from my lungs. I tried to inhale, but even that was nearly impossible.

Frustration turned to panic. I was trapped in a truck leaking gasoline on a remote country road late at night, unable to shout or even breathe, and nobody knew it. The accident happened less than a mile from home, but the distance suddenly felt infinite.

I'd just dropped off my girlfriend at her house. We were excited about the junior prom that was a few weeks away. We were talking about a future that glowed with romance and possibilities. I was 17. I had my whole life ahead of me. Now I was about to die alone, in the dark, my charred body to be discovered hours later in the blackened hulk of the pickup, most likely by my poor father who would go looking for me when I failed to come home on time.

If I could have, I would have sobbed. Instead, I prayed.

HOW I ROLL

*life, love, & work
after a spinal
cord injury*

1
farm boy

You might say, in spite of what happened, that I've been lucky in life. As a youngster and young adult, my ambitions were modest. Getting rich, being famous, living an exotic life doing something dangerous or fascinating—none of that held the allure of following in the path of my parents: I wanted to work hard, marry a nice girl, and raise healthy, happy children.

My modest ambitions may have made my life's journey a little easier than if I had had loftier goals. Although nothing can prepare a person for what I have experienced, I think it helped to have grown up in a community where people instinctively looked out for each other. Many people have looked out for me, and I doubt I could have achieved what I have without them.

I grew up in DeWitt, a small town in Dinwiddie County, Virginia, where most of the folks I knew lived on small family farms surrounded by acres of tobacco, wheat, and soybeans. Dinwiddie County is only an hour from the state capital in Richmond and two hours from the busy port of Norfolk at the mouth of the Chesapeake

— ⚡ —

Bay.

My parents, James, Sr. and Gloria, both grew up on farms in Dinwiddie. My father's family raised livestock and grew tobacco, and my mother's family had a dairy farm. As teenagers, Dad played baseball and Mom played basketball. They met at each other's high school sporting events, the main social venue for teens.

Mom went on to Radford College, about four hours away, studying to become a teacher. She lived in a dorm, and came home occasionally on weekends. During one of those visits in her sophomore year, she happened to be closest to the phone when it rang and she answered.

"Hello, this is Jimmy Neville," a young voice blurted. "I met you at a basketball game and I wonder if you'd like to go out sometime."

"Sure!"

After they'd made plans, my mother hung up, turned to her sister, Carol, also a former high school basketball player, and announced, "One of us has a date with Jimmy Neville, but I'm not sure which!" Since my mother had answered the phone and made the plans, she claimed the date. It must have been love at first sight for them both because they immediately became a couple and were married in July of 1962, after my mother had earned her BA and teaching certificate.

I showed up the next year, on October 24, 1963. I was named James, Jr., so to avoid confusion my parents called me by my middle name, Bryant. There was only one doctor in DeWitt and my arrival proved inconvenient for W. W. Howard, an older man whose hernia operation was delayed while the doctor delivered me. I can remember old Mr. Howard teasing me when he saw me around town. "You know you nearly killed me, making me wait for my operation!"

My mother taught second grade first at Dinwiddie Elementary and later at South Side Elementary. My father repaired tires at a local tire store. Later he operated a bulldozer, worked as a mechanic in the school bus garage, and finally got a job at Continental Forest Industries, a local sawmill that produced lumber, mulch, and paper pulp. He worked his way up to plant manager before retiring to work as a general contractor.

For the first eight years of my life, we lived in modest rented houses while my parents planned to build a house on a plot of land on my grandfather Neville's farm. Our final rented house was shabby and the plaster walls were webbed with so many cracks we joked that we had air conditioning and heating—keeping us cold in the winter and hot in the summer. We took our circumstances in stride, because we knew our permanent home was nearing completion.

In 1972, we moved into our brand-new house on the farm, the same house my parents live in today, a modest two-bedroom with a pond out back and lots of room for me to play and explore.

Grandfather Neville—who we called Papa—helped my father build our house. He was a master plumber and electrician who never turned down a job if his customer couldn't pay. Papa worked hard his whole life. Just before we moved into our house, he came home from cutting the grass at the church, sat down to rest, and had a fatal heart attack.

A hat he'd hung on a valve of the hot water furnace in the basement of our new home stayed there undisturbed for the next 38 years, until the old furnace was replaced. If the hat hadn't fallen apart, my parents would have put it on the new heater. Gestures like that—honoring family and values—left a big impression on me.

When Mom returned to work after my birth, she dropped me off at the home of Dad's cousin Ray, where I stayed with his wife, Brenda, and their three young children. When Brenda returned to work a couple of years later, I stayed with Mom's mother, Grandma Patsy. She was my favorite playmate, and for many years I was her only grandchild.

Grandma made me pancakes every day for breakfast. While she tidied the kitchen, I watched my favorite shows on tv: *Sailor Bob, Gilligan's Island, The Beverly Hillbillies*, or *The Andy Griffith Show*. Mid-mornings and afternoons were spent playing, but everything came to a halt midday when her soaps came on TV and I had to be on my best behavior.

A few years after I was born, my mother started feeling unwell and was diagnosed with diabetes insipidus, a disease affecting the pituitary. The doctor told her the medication she needed to live would make another pregnancy dangerous and she should avoid trying to have more children.

I may have been an only child but I never lacked companionship. My father's brother Tom had two sons: Johnny was two years older and Steve was just six months older. They lived half a mile away, so the three of us grew up as close as brothers.

Johnny was husky and Steve was rail-thin. They often got into fierce scraps, Steve grabbing a stick or a rock to even the odds until Johnny one-upped him with a bigger stick or rock. I stayed out of harm's way on the sidelines. I never wanted to get caught misbehaving, because the punishment was swift and consistent. You'd get a spanking from whoever caught you, be it a parent, relative, or unrelated adult at church or school.

In spite of all their fighting, let anyone threaten Johnny or Steve and the other one immediately came to his defense. It was one of my first lessons in family loyalty.

Staying out of trouble wasn't that hard once I started pitching in with the chores around our house and on the farm, like weeding the garden, feeding the animals, mowing the grass, and chopping firewood. Everything was done by hand. The whole family spent June to September raising and harvesting tobacco. Even the youngest of us helped, handing pulled leaves to the adults who tied them into bunches for drying.

In winter, the family gathered for the annual hog butchering. This was the source of much of our food supply—sausage, ham, pork chops, bacon, and lard. Frugal farm families used every part of the pig, even the intestines, which were washed and fried, served as chitterlings, or "chittlins"—considered by some a Southern delicacy. Not me—I couldn't get over the fact that they were pigs' guts and was glad no one forced me to eat them.

Back then we didn't have a profusion of supermarkets and convenience stores, so neighbors traded what they grew or raised with each other. Outings to one of the two closest market towns, Blackstone or Petersburg, only happened around the tobacco harvest and at Christmas, when Dad gave me a few dollars to buy

Christmas presents. In between, we made things last. Most of us kids went barefoot in the summer to keep from wearing out our shoes.

I was apprehensive about leaving Grandma Patsy's for first grade at Dinwiddie Elementary, where my mother taught. I took one look at the classroom of 30 other children and ran to my mother's classroom door in tears. This went on for several days until I overcame my shyness and realized school was fun. I came to love my teachers, classes, and classmates and brought home straight A's in every subject except band, where my mediocre saxophone skills earned me a B.

There was only one after-school activity: baseball. Kids were either in Peewee League, Little League, or Pony League, but baseball it was. Even our fathers played baseball in the Virginia League, and my lifelong love of the game was born watching Dad play.

Dinwiddie felt far away from the political turmoil of the day—the Cold War, the Vietnam War, the moon landing, Watergate. Folks were more worried about getting by than politics—in my family we watched sitcoms instead of the news. My knowledge of war was confined to the escapades of the doctors on *M*A*S*H* and my distaste for prejudice was informed by the awkwardly hilarious bigotry of Archie Bunker on *All in the Family*. The Fonz on *Happy Days* was my definition of cool.

For summer vacations, we'd pile into the car with Dad's sisters Nancy and Glenice and their families and drive to North Carolina to attractions like Grandfather Mountain State Park or Tweetsie Railroad, a Wild West theme park, spending a few days in a motel.

After a few years, the big family vacations ceased

and my parents sent me to spend a week every summer with my Aunt Carol and her husband, Bill. They lived in Midlothian, a suburb on the western outskirts of Richmond. We played putt-putt golf, got Big Macs from McDonald's, went to the movies, and swam in her neighbor's pool. These were all things I couldn't do

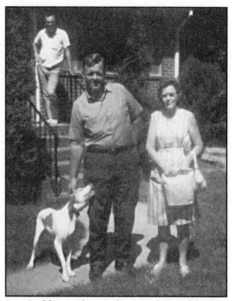

Big Daddy taught me how to hunt, fish, and appreciate life. Grandma Patsy was one of my first playmates.

in rural DeWitt, and I loved every minute of my stay.

As I grew older, I became close with my mother's father, who we called Big Daddy. Big Daddy worked at a rock quarry and was broad and stood 6'6" tall. He was strong enough to carry a full ten-gallon milk can in each hand and lift both onto the truck at the same time without spilling a drop. He was kind and loving—a gentle giant.

On summer Saturdays we went fishing. He came over around 3:30 in the morning, hollering, "You going to sleep all day or are we going fishing?" I've been an early riser ever since.

Big Daddy was the best fly fisher I've ever seen, getting his line into impossibly tight spots. I'd try to do the same and often got my line caught in the trees or bushes. Big Daddy would laugh and catch a few more fish before helping me get untangled. Those mornings taught me the value of patience.

We fished until about 10 or 11, when it got too hot for the fish to bite, and then went to a local hunt club where the men played a card game called Setback. These men never drank or gambled—that crowd arrived after we left—but they did tell tall tales, repeated week after week. I never tired of hearing them. With each retelling, the details grew more outrageous.

During the rest of the year, we hunted whatever was in season. When I was ten I got my first gun—a 20-gauge single barrel shotgun. Big Daddy rounded up his bird dogs and taught me to shoot doves and quail before moving on to bigger game. We hunted deer from October to January. Whatever we caught or shot came home with us for food—we hunted and fished for fun, but we didn't waste a thing.

One December day when I was 13, Big Daddy and I were hunting deer along an old fire road. A small buck bolted out of the woods a few feet from me. I was startled and fired three times, all misses. Embarrassed, I walked down the road toward Big Daddy, who stood about a hundred yards away. I expected him to tease me, but instead, he quietly said, "Bryant, look up."

The end of the tree branch a few inches above his head was snapped off. "Now look down here," he said, pointing just beyond his feet to a spot where the dirt had been stirred up. My legs turned to jelly, and I felt numb with shock. In my haste to shoot the deer, I'd nearly shot my grandfather.

The gun dropped from my hands as I threw my arms around Big Daddy's neck to keep myself from falling. What if I'd killed him? Instead of scolding me, Big Daddy wrapped me in his arms and said, "This is something you'll never forget, son. The way you've learned this lesson will never leave you." He was right. From then on, I became a vigilant and careful hunter.

On Sundays we went to church. My parents had attended different churches and when they married, rather than choose one over the other, they compromised and chose a new one in DeWitt: Bott Memorial Presbyterian Church. Like most country churches, it had a small congregation of about 60 members.

After church services, Dad's five brothers and sisters and their spouses and children gathered at Grandma Neville's for a big midday meal. Grandma always served meatloaf or one of my favorites, fried chicken, with mashed potatoes, biscuits, and gravy. Then we'd go to Grandma Patsy and Big Daddy's to play pinochle or rummy and have dinner, which always included creamed vegetable dishes and milk gravy made with milk from their dairy.

My childhood was modest, but I was happy and secure in my family's love. My parents had rules I was expected to follow, but they were loving and involved, meeting my friends, helping with my schoolwork, and watching my baseball games. We had dinner together every night and did everything together as a family. If they were invited someplace I couldn't go to, they usually didn't go either.

From a young age, I knew I wanted to grow up and become as good a husband and as loving a father as Dad.

2
a girlfriend and a car

When I started eighth grade at Dinwiddie Junior High School, my focus shifted from academics to my social life, and by the time I started tenth grade at Dinwiddie High, my glowing report cards were history. I was one of the first tenth graders to get my driver's license—my October birthday meant I'd started school a year later than my classmates, so I was a year older than them. Mixing girls and driving was the downfall of my education.

I made three new friends: Jamie Kennedy, Walter Wells, and my best friend, Jimmy Stidham. We did everything together. Jimmy was originally from the hills of Norton, Virginia, just east of the West Virginia line. He was small and wiry compared to my husky 6'4" frame, and he had fire-engine-red hair and a temper to match. Jamie was the fifth in a line of six boys, followed by one little sister. He grew up on a farm and all the hard work, done by hand, made him rail thin. Walter and I had been in school together since second grade but only got to know each other as teens. He was tall—just over six feet—but also quite thin. We were different as could be but were as close as brothers.

We loved going to the bowling alley or the pool hall in Petersburg, which also had video games and darts and was a popular gathering place for our classmates. I was big for my age, so I could get away with buying beer. We never got into any serious trouble, but we certainly weren't saints.

Jimmy's short temper got him into his fair share of fights, and he was quick to throw punches at anyone who insulted him or his friends. One night at the pool hall parking lot, I found Jimmy preparing to fight a stranger—why I don't know. By now the guy's friends were rallying around him, among them a huge, angry guy whose face was covered in scars. This was clearly someone used to swinging his fists—possibly even weapons. My heart started pounding. I wanted to run back into the pool hall, but I wouldn't abandon my friend.

The huge guy turned to me and snarled, "Y'all don't mess with my brothers."

I tried hard to look brave and said, "Well, don't mess with mine."

I'm not sure what made the fight go out of him, but he walked away and I felt weak with relief. Thank you, Lord, I silently prayed. I was certain that if we had gotten into a fight, this man could have seriously hurt me— maybe even killed me. The other guys walked away too, without throwing a single punch. We were lucky to avoid a physical confrontation that night, but I knew if I'd had to fight, I would have given it my all. I'd meant what I'd said: my friends were like brothers, and I always stuck up for my family.

The summer after tenth grade, I started working with my Uncle Billy. He was my dad's youngest brother and only eleven years older than me, so he was pretty cool to hang out with. He did plumbing and electrical work, and together we responded to service calls about leaks and stopped-up drains. It was my first paying job—my chores were considered par for the course—and it was gratifying to see those hours of hard work amount to a regular paycheck. My spending money let me spring for things like beer and rounds of pool and bowling, which made me quite popular.

By this point my grades were mostly C's and D's. The only class I liked was automotive shop. I didn't have plans to become a mechanic, but I enjoyed a break from the books. The shop teacher, who we called Doc Evans, was particularly fond of me because I could drive and run errands for him. Sometimes these took so long that I missed later classes—usually Mrs. Bolte's English class. She was my Sunday school teacher's wife, so I saw her regularly, and she always gave me grief about missing her class. I was also a member of the Future Farmers of America club in junior high and high school—mostly because it meant getting out of class.

My parents never got on my case about my poor grades, but I'm sure they wished I could have kept up the straight A's and gone to college. I wasn't interested—more years in a classroom weren't appealing. I wanted a job that didn't require a fancy degree but that would make me lots of money, even though I wasn't particularly motivated to work hard for it. If all else failed, I could get a job in agriculture or doing manual labor. So I coasted along with a vague sense that I'd figure out what to do when the time came.

In the spring of 1979, Big Daddy started feeling unwell. He got tired more quickly and had frequent indigestion and stomach pain. His physician thought he was developing an ulcer and prescribed antacids, but these didn't help. Soon the smallest task exhausted him, and his stomach pain grew worse. In late May, Big Daddy underwent exploratory surgery that had a grim diagnosis: stomach cancer.

This shook my faith. How could such a kind and gentle man be dealt such a raw hand? I was terrified of losing him. My fear reminded me of my childhood near-miss with the gun. I had nearly lost Big Daddy then but had learned that being careful would prevent a future tragedy. But now there was nothing I could do—the situation was out of my control. I did my best to wear a brave face and stay positive, but inside I felt like I was dying right along with him.

The doctor ordered chemotherapy that took place five days a week at MCV Hospital in Richmond. I had my learner's permit—in Virginia, we were allowed to get one at age 15 years and 8 months—and school was out for the summer, so I took on the responsibility of driving him back and forth to his treatments in his Dodge Dart.

My careful driving impressed Big Daddy. "I can't wait to see you get that license," he told me.

"Don't worry, Big Daddy. I'm taking the test in October. You'll be the first to see it." I didn't say what I was thinking: that I hoped he'd be alive to see it.

— ⚡ —

We had many conversations that summer. Some were retellings of favorite tales we'd shared over the years while others were new. Big Daddy always steered our talks toward a lesson he wanted me to learn. He seemed to know his days were numbered and wanted to prepare me to face the world without him. His most important lesson was about trust and honor.

"Bryant, trust and honor are two different things, but they are interconnected and they are both equally important. Do you understand the difference?"

I thought for a moment. "Now that I think about it, I'm not sure that I do."

"Trust is the belief others have in you when they know they can rely on you. You have to earn it, and it's very hard or impossible to get it back if it's broken, so you must always be honest. Honor is you knowing that the trust others have in you is well deserved. It's what lets you go to sleep at night happy in the knowledge that you are an honest man true to his word and worthy of trust."

He let it sink in for a minute, then added, "A good way to sum this up is: always do what you say and say what you do, son."

"I will, Big Daddy, I promise."

My beloved grandfather succumbed quickly to his illness. Over the summer he grew weaker and more uncomfortable until he was hospitalized. Soon he was jaundiced and seemed unaware of his surroundings. It was devastating to see this strong, tall man who had taught me to fish and hunt become a shell of his former self. He'd always been there for me, and I suppose I believed he always would be.

I was still determined to show him my driver's

⚡
---

license, so when I passed the test in October, I drove straight to the hospital to show it to him.

His eyes were closed. "Hey, Big Daddy," I said. "It's me, Bryant. Look." I held up the card. "I got my license."

As I approached his bed, his eyes were closed. "Big Daddy," I said softly. "I have something to show you."

He opened his eyes and looked at me. I wasn't sure he recognized me, so I said, "Hey, Big Daddy. It's me, Bryant. Look." I held up the card. "I got my license."

I believe that he knew what it was and think that even in his silence, he was proud. That evening, Big Daddy died.

I'd stayed brave and positive during Big Daddy's illness, but at this point, I shut down. One of the two most important men in life was gone, and nothing seemed important anymore. I lost interest in my usual pastimes, even hunting and fishing. I didn't feel anger or disbelief. I was just numb. Most of the time, I felt like finding a place to hide from life.

After several months, my Uncle Billy intervened. One day in early spring we were together at our hunt club. Big Daddy had loved being at the club, and his absence was a huge weight on my shoulders. Billy noticed I was withdrawn and pulled me aside.

"Bryant, I've watched your attitude go south for a while. What's going on?"

I shrugged. "I don't know."

"I do, and so does everybody else," he said sternly.

"Look Bryant, I know you're still upset about Big Daddy and that you miss him, but you need to understand that no one is happy about what happened. You're not the only one who misses him. He was good to all of us."

I looked at him sullenly.

"Bryant, you need to move on. Big Daddy wouldn't be happy seeing you mope around like this. It's not helping anyone or anything. You need to get your head out of your ass and realize that the people we love die, and you need to get on with your life."

The painful words Billy bravely said were what I'd long needed to hear: Big Daddy would have hated seeing me miserable. The best way to honor his memory was to get back into my life. It wasn't easy, but soon I found myself fully engrossed in my friendships, my fishing rod and shotgun, and my summer job with Billy. I still missed Big Daddy terribly, but knowing he was in Heaven free of his painful illness and watching out for me restored my faith. I'm sure that chat has long since left Billy's memory, but I will never forget how he helped me.

My parents must have noticed the change in my behavior, because they offered to help me buy a car of my own: a candy-apple-red 1973 Dodge Challenger. I also had to pay for gas and maintenance, a responsibility I gladly accepted because my treasured car gave me independence. It had a high-performance 340-cubic-inch Hemi engine and a sweet-sounding four-barrel carburetor. It was a gem of a car—I was very proud of it and took great care of it.

Having my own car further boosted my popularity, and my social life was booming. For a while I had lots of different girlfriends without committing to any of them for very long. Then Amy Livingston came along and changed everything.

Amy was different from the other girls I'd dated. We had known each other since junior high and started spending time together in high school. By my junior year, we were an item. We were so compatible that I lost interest in dating other girls and was content to be with just her. She got along with my friends and was caring and fun loving. Amy was tall and slim, with curves in all the right places. She had dark brown curly hair, hazel eyes, and a beautiful smile. There was something special about her that made me never want to leave her side. It didn't matter where we went or what we did as long as we were together.

By spring of my junior year, I seemed to have it all: a steady girlfriend, a great group of friends, a car, and my own spending money. Amy and I made plans to go to our junior prom in April. Our friends were attending and we looked forward to a special night together. One Saturday in March, we decided to go get my prom tux fitted.

Life was good again.

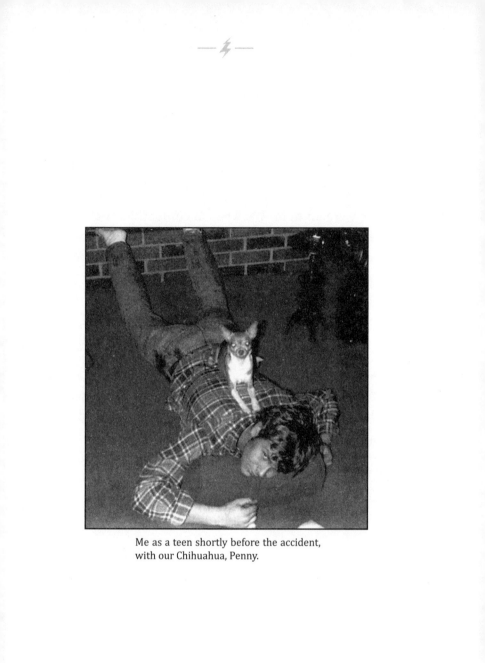

Me as a teen shortly before the accident,
with our Chihuahua, Penny.

3
losing control

On the evening of Saturday, March 21, Amy and I went to a local formalwear shop where I was fitted for my rental tuxedo. It was an exciting time, because we also got our class rings.

Afterward, we drove over to Petersburg to the bowling alley and spent the rest of the evening with our friends.

I had to get Amy home for her 11 o'clock curfew. That night I'd taken my dad's pickup truck—a small four-cylinder Dodge D50 Ram—instead of my own Dodge Challenger. I had two reasons for my vehicle choice. First, economics: I was driving more than usual that night and his truck got better gas mileage. Second, hormonal: my car's sporty bucket seats were no match for the pickup's long front seat, which made it easy to cozy up to Amy for an abundance of goodnight kisses.

After leaving a thoroughly kissed Amy at her house, I started for home. My stomach rumbled—between the fitting and meeting our friends, we hadn't eaten dinner.

I pulled into a fast food joint to have a burger before continuing home.

It was about midnight when I finally got onto Route 645, the road our house was on. I had to travel three miles of desolate country road, where the houses were spread out and there were no streetlights. I was full from my late-night snack and yawned as I steered down the dark road. Climbing into bed would feel good.

I approached the final curve before the road became a straight one-mile shot to my house. As I rounded the curve, something glimmered in the headlights, and my drowsy brain took a second to realize it was a deer in the road. I turned the wheel sharply to drive around the deer and the truck started to skid onto the shoulder. To correct the turn, I yanked the wheel hard in the other direction. This tactic would have worked in my car, which was heavy and low to the ground, but it was a bad move in my father's lightweight pickup. The truck teetered back up onto the asphalt and went into a roll as I clung desperately to the steering wheel.

It took just a few seconds for the truck to roll across our two-lane country road, but I felt like I was tumbling over and over for days. In 1981, there was no seatbelt law and many people didn't wear them. I hadn't fastened mine, so I was tossed around the truck's cab and my head smashed into the top of the passenger doorframe.

The truck came to a stop against a clump of three small trees on the other side of the road. It was completely dark and silent—I couldn't see a single star or hear a single insect or animal. I was enveloped by nothingness. Was I dead?

After a few dazed moments, the truck's interior

came into focus and I realized that I was still alive. The truck was upside down and I was slumped against the smashed passenger window, my head in the grass on the roadside. The headlights were the only light piercing the darkness.

> The truck's interior came into focus and I realized that I was still alive.

The smell of gas filled my nostrils, and I realized it was leaking from the truck. Television car explosions replayed themselves in my head—what if the same thing happened to the pickup? I had to get out of there.

I tried to wriggle out of the cab through the window but couldn't move. I was in an awkward position and figured my legs were stuck, so I tried to shake them free. Nothing happened. Then I tried moving my arms, but again, nothing happened and I realized they must be pinned down. What was going on? Was I trapped? I felt the first prickles of panic.

Even though it was difficult, I could still move my head, so I thrashed it around, figuring that the motion would free me from the wreckage. I heard a clicking sound like pool balls striking each other, which I thought was my body shaking loose, but I quickly realized I was still in the same position. I was trapped.

Panic spread through my body. I knew it was a long shot, since the closest house wasn't near the roadside, but I decided to yell for help. Hopefully my voice would carry through the quiet night and someone would hear. I opened my mouth to yell and nothing came out.

Take a deep breath, Bryant, I told myself. Calm down then yell at the top of your lungs. But the problem *was* my lungs. I couldn't take a deep breath or get air into my body. It felt like it was leaking out of me. Suddenly, yelling a one-syllable word was impossible.

I couldn't move. I couldn't yell. I could barely even breathe. I was trapped upside-down in a wrecked truck that was leaking gas on a dark, infrequently traveled road. I could see no way out of a seemingly certain death sentence. I couldn't even feel any pain. All I felt was terror so strong it numbed everything else. I couldn't believe I was mere moments from what would surely be an excruciating death. I imagined my friends and family at my funeral—my father comforting my sobbing mother, Jimmy and Jamie and Walter looking grim, Amy's silent tears—and wondered what awaited me in the afterlife. Would Big Daddy and Papa be waiting there for me?

There was nothing else I could do, so I started to silently pray. "Dear God, I don't want to die. I tried to be a good person, a good son and friend. I don't want to burn up and suffer. Please help me."

A feeling of intense peace suddenly settled over me, like a wave pushing away the terror. I could hear Big Daddy's voice inside my head saying, "Don't worry, son. It's going to be okay. I won't leave you. Hang in there. You'll be all right."

It was like his words flipped a switch. The seemingly silent night was suddenly alive with noises again— crickets and frogs and nocturnal animals making their rounds. The pitch-black sky I could see through the cracked windshield was now dotted with hundreds of stars. I could feel the chill of the night air on my face. The smell of gas, the only thing I had been focusing on,

—⚡—

grew fainter. Big Daddy's presence comforted me. I lay in peace for several minutes.

I detected a faint sound and strained to hear it. It grew louder and I realized it was a car coming toward me. I heard it stop a few feet away and tried to holler.

Footsteps pounded over to the side of the truck where I lay. A familiar voice shouted, "Bryant! Bryant, is that you?" It was my cousin Steve, coming home from a night out. It was past his curfew and I silently thanked God that he was late.

I tried to reply, but Steve said, "Hold on, Bryant, I'm going to get help. Hold on!" He raced back to his car and sped off to his parents' house. I closed my eyes in relief.

The next thing I knew, I awoke to the sound of sirens approaching. I had blacked out. There were police and paramedics milling around, and my parents were among the throng of people. The paramedics talked to me as they loaded me onto a stretcher and into an ambulance, but I was fading in and out of consciousness and couldn't focus on their words. They fitted a brace around my neck and examined my head. I still couldn't feel my arms or legs and was unable to speak but was relieved that help had arrived.

The ambulance sped up Interstate 85 to Petersburg General Hospital, my parents following in their car. From the stretcher I couldn't see much out the windows, but I noticed that

I couldn't see much out the windows, but I noticed that we sped through the tollbooth without stopping.

we sped through the tollbooth without stopping. It felt like we were going about a hundred miles an hour.

Big Daddy had been right. I had held on, and I was okay. I could no longer hear his voice but I could still feel his presence. I said a silent prayer of thanks before I blacked out.

4
lightning strikes

When I finally came to, it took me a few moments to realize that I was in a cold, bright emergency room mobbed with doctors and nurses. I was still wearing the neck brace, and my whole head throbbed, especially at the top and back. A nurse stood where I could see her.

"Bryant, there's a large wound in your head that we need to clean up and stitch," she explained. "We don't know where else you're injured, so we can't give you any anesthesia. It's going to hurt, so I'm giving you this to bite on." She placed what felt like a stick between my teeth.

First the nurses had to cut my hair from around the wound. My dark blond hair wasn't long, but it was thick and curled around my ears and the base of my neck. The dried blood around the wound made it difficult to remove the hair, and I seemed to feel each strand being torn away from the gash. Then the nurses washed and disinfected the wound with what felt like a mixture of alcohol and gasoline—my skin was on fire! But the worst was yet to come.

As the doctor began to suture my wound, each stitch hurt worse than the last, and I'll never know how I managed not to bite clear through that stick. The gash was long, running from the center of my head back toward my neck, so it required many stitches that seemed to take ages. I don't remember the nurse removing the stick from my mouth because my head rang with pain that blotted out everything else. With every heartbeat, the stitches throbbed. I'm convinced that I swallowed that stick.

After this torture, I mercifully spent most of the time they were administering tests, X-rays, and scans out of consciousness. When I awoke, I was in a room in the intensive care unit, my parents anxiously hovering nearby.

"Bryant!" my mother cried. "Oh, Bryant, I'm so glad you're awake." Seeing two familiar faces after the swarm of doctors and nurses was comforting.

"How are you feeling, son?" my dad asked.

"Okay," I managed to croak. "My head hurts. It's sort of hard to breathe. Mom, Dad, what's wrong with me? What did they say?"

"We don't know yet, honey," my mother said. "We should hear from the doctor tomorrow. Now get some rest. We'll be here with you, don't worry."

The next day, a doctor came to speak with us. "Bryant has broken several cervical vertebrae high up in his spinal cord," he told us. I remembered the clicking sound when I'd thrashed my head. With a chill, I realized it was the sound of my broken neck bones striking each other.

"We're going to perform an operation where we take a piece of bone from his hip and fuse it into his neck to help stabilize it," the doctor explained. "To do this, we're first going to put Bryant in traction."

I couldn't eat or drink. I longed to sink my teeth into a steak.

"Sounds fun," I rasped.

The doctor continued. "We'll put a halo on his head and use that to stretch out his neck so we can better perform the surgery."

I was wary about the stretching part but figured it couldn't be that bad—haloes are angelic headwear, after all.

It was anything but heavenly. The doctors had to affix the metal ring to my head using small screws that went into my skull. That was agonizing—the screws weren't enormous, but they felt like giant spikes. Then the doctors attached what they claimed was a small weight to the halo to help with the stretching. It felt like a hundred pounds.

At this point, I still couldn't feel my arms or legs, and I was declared NPO—an abbreviation for the Latin phrase *nil per os*—which meant I couldn't eat or drink anything. I was fed intravenously, and occasionally a nurse would wipe an ice cube wrapped in a washcloth over my parched lips, but I longed to sink my teeth into something like a steak.

The night before my surgery, my exhausted parents, who had been living between my room and the ICU waiting room, finally went home to sleep. The nurses left a call button on my pillow that I could press by slightly moving my head. As the hours passed, it became harder to take breaths and I frantically pressed the button.

I liked most everyone on the staff, but the night nurse was not pleasant. "What?" she snapped.

"Please," I gasped. "I can't breathe. Please call my parents."

"You'll be fine," she said dismissively. "Quit bothering me. Go back to sleep." She left.

I tried my best to relax, but it was so hard to breathe that I couldn't. After a while, I called her again. Again she came in, looking mightily annoyed. Again she told me to stop worrying and left without helping me.

As I lay there alone, convinced this was my last night on earth, I had a silent talk with the Man upstairs. "God, if this is my time to go, then let's go. I've suffered enough already and I don't want to suffer anymore. I don't want to die, but if now's the time, I just want to go. I can't deal with much more of this. If there's more I'm meant to do here and this isn't my time, please give me the strength to cope, God. Help me understand Your plan for me."

After my prayer, I figured I'd try one last time to get help. I paged the nurse a third time, and miraculously, she begrudgingly agreed to call my parents and get me help. After my father arrived and found out what happened, I never saw her again.

It was comforting to have Mom and Dad with me, but it wasn't any easier to breathe. The cold night air on the night of the accident coupled with my now-diminished lung capacity had caused pneumonia. The first and second vertebrae control functions necessary to live, including lung control for breathing. My injury occurred in the third through fifth vertebrae, which meant I could breathe on my own, but it affected the muscles in and around my chest and abdomen. This made actions like coughing or yelling nearly impossible. The thick mucus caused by my pneumonia was filling my lungs but I couldn't cough to clear it.

I believed the pneumonia was God's way of granting my prayer for relief and I thought I was close to death. Part of me welcomed an escape from my suffering, but I wasn't quite ready to go. It was scary to think of leaving my parents and the life I loved. I was exhausted but fought my body's urge to sleep, convinced that closing my eyes and nodding off meant I'd die.

As I struggled to keep my eyes open, I once again heard Big Daddy's voice. "It's all right, Bryant. You just go to sleep and rest. I'm with you, you'll be okay." The quiet and darkness that had moments before terrified me now seemed peaceful and inviting. I knew Big Daddy would keep me safe, just as he had in the truck's wreckage, and let my eyelids shut. The next thing I knew, it was morning and I was alive.

The doctors planned to put in a respirator during my surgery to help me breathe. They were also going to perform a tracheotomy and insert a suction tube to clear the mucus from my lungs. I figured my numerous procedures were monopolizing half the equipment in the hospital, but I knew it would be worth it when I could move again.

When I awoke from the surgery hours later, the respirator and trach tube were in my throat. This made it impossible to speak so I had to mouth everything, but at least I could breathe!

Soon after the respirator was put in, I was lying in my room conversing with my father—he speaking, I mouthing back—when everything went black. My panicked father ran to get help and I awoke, dazed, to find Mike, one of the ICU nurses, straddling me and pounding on my chest. What had just happened?

"Your heart stopped," Mike said. Oh boy, I thought. Would I constantly be teetering on the brink of death?

A doctor hurried in and after examining my chart explained, "Bryant, your body is full of different medications and there's not enough liquid in your body to absorb them properly. The doses were potent enough to stop your heart. We'll adjust your medication so this won't happen again." Thankfully he was right. I didn't think I could take one more terrifying near-death escape.

In my moments alone in the ICU, I reflected on what had happened to me. Surviving several terrifying brushes with death shook my faith. My life had been spared more than once, but at the cost of great suffering to me and my family. I had asked God to help me understand His plan for me, but so far it just looked like I was meant to deal with one medical drama after another. What had I done to deserve this? Maybe I got into a little trouble with my friends sometimes, and I wasn't the greatest student, but I was a good son, friend, and boyfriend. Why had that deer appeared? Why hadn't I worn a seatbelt? Why had this happened to me? I was deeply discouraged and angry.

The next afternoon, my mother excitedly told me, "Bryant, I'm sure you're too far away to have heard this, but earlier today there was a single clap of thunder near our house."

"That's weird," I mouthed back. Thunderstorms in March were scarce in central Virginia.

"Well, it was really loud, so we knew the lightning had struck close to the house. We went out to look around," she continued. Her expression was one of awe as she told me, "The lightning struck the tree where Dad's truck stopped on the night of your accident.

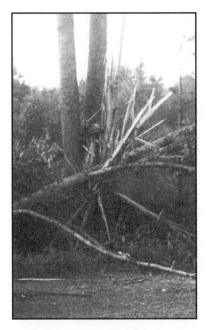

The tree I hit was blasted a few days later by a rare March lightning strike. The other two trees next to it were untouched.

There are three trees growing close together there, but Dad's truck touched only one of them, and that's the only one that was destroyed."

"Blown to splinters," Dad said.

I felt a chill. How had this single lightning strike, such a rare occurrence in early spring, happened to destroy only the tree the truck had touched on the night of my accident, leaving the other two trees untouched? This was God's answer to my prayer, exactly what I needed to hear to restore my faith. The lightning strike proved that my life had purpose and meaning—I just had to be confident and trust that I would learn God's plan for me in good time. I could have died in the ICU, or the night of the accident, but I didn't. I must have survived for a reason, and now that I'd gotten this second chance, I wouldn't waste it. My determination to get better grew stronger each day.

Seeing my family and friends helped strengthen my resolve. It seemed like almost everyone I knew came to visit me in the ICU. The ICU had a strict immediate-family-only policy, but my nurses knew visitors were better than any medicine, so they bent the rules. My grandmothers, aunts, uncles, and cousins came, as well as my friends and even a few of my teachers, including my shop teacher, Doc Evans. He was a black man, and when they asked how he was related to me, he replied, "I'm the black sheep of the family." This was obviously the right answer, because they let him in.

It was especially wonderful to see Amy. She sat by my bed and held my hand, lifting it up so I could see it since I still hadn't regained any feeling in my limbs. During one of her visits, I told her, "I don't think I'll be going to prom."

"I won't go either," she said. "I don't want to go without you."

"No way," I protested. "You can't miss prom." I decided that my father would escort her for the evening. This way she could still go to the prom, and I could be sure her date wouldn't threaten my position as her boyfriend.

After two and a half weeks in intensive care, the doctors determined that they could safely remove the respirator, although they would leave the trach in to continue clearing my lung congestion. I had been under anesthesia when they'd put in the respirator, but I was awake for its removal. It felt like a bowling ball was being pulled out of my lungs and throat and through my nose. When the nurse showed me the tube, I protested, "That's not what came out of my nose. It felt a hundred times bigger."

It felt a bowling ball was being pulled out of my lungs and throat through my nose.

Now that the respirator was gone, I was moved to the progressive care wing for a week. The NPO order was lifted and I was allowed to have food and drink again. One of my favorite nurses, Dot, brought me a can of 7-Up soda. She held the straw to my mouth and I took a long, satisfying drink. It was the greatest thing I'd ever tasted.

In addition to real food, progressive care also meant longer visiting hours, and my visitors were eager to bring me treats. One of the first things I craved was banana popsicles. These were challenging to find, but my family fanned out and combed the area. My Aunt Betty found a 7-11 convenience store that carried them and bought me a stockpile. My dad's boss also made me an amazing steak and delivered it to the hospital. The food my family brought me far surpassed anything from the cafeteria, and I ate like a king.

I needed to be fed these treats, since I was still immobile from the neck down. I also had a low-grade fever, due to a bladder infection, and was on a special mattress that circulated cold water to try and keep me cool. The doctors still hadn't given me a definitive long-term diagnosis. They had explained that the break in my neck had caused paralysis in my arms and legs, but they didn't explain just how long I could expect this to last. I assumed that once my spinal cord injury healed, I'd be walking again.

Soon I'd be leaving for a rehabilitation center, where I'd receive lots of physical therapy to relearn how to use my limbs. My family and I noticed that my legs had started randomly moving on their own—a good sign.

"Let's make sure we tell the neurologist about this," I told my parents. "It's got to mean that I'm getting better." The neurologist was due to check in with us one last time before we left for rehab, and I was hoping he'd give us good news.

Visits with Amy were often bittersweet. I loved seeing her, but I also felt like I was holding her back and I knew it would be hard to stay together while I was away at rehab. We had some serious talks about our future together.

"Amy, I really think you should consider seeing other people," I finally told her.

She took my hand. "Bryant, what are you talking about? I'm not interested in seeing other people. I'm with you, and I want to stay with you."

She wasn't making this any easier! I took a deep breath and pressed on.

"I have no idea what's going to happen to me. I might get better and be able to leave rehab pretty quickly, or I might be there for a while. I don't want you to put your life on hold for me while I'm away."

I swallowed the lump in my throat. "This is my road to go down, I don't want to drag you along with me."

"Bryant." She shook her head. "I want to go down that road with you! I want to be there to support you. I know it'll be hard, and we'll be far apart, but we can visit and talk on the phone. I'm not going to give up on you, or us, just because of this." She smiled. I couldn't imagine a more loyal or loving girlfriend and I felt like the luckiest guy on earth.

"I know it'll be hard, but I'm not going to give up on you, or us, just because of this."

"Okay," I finally agreed. "I'll work twice as hard to get better so I can come back home sooner." What better motivation could there be?

I was going to Woodrow Wilson Rehabilitation Center, located a four-hour drive away in Fishersville. I would fly there in a small plane, which was both exciting and nerve-racking because I'd never flown before.

My mother quit her teaching job so she could stay near the center and see me each day, and Grandma Neville was coming too. My father had to stay home to work, but he promised to visit as often as he could, as did my other relatives, my friends, and Amy, which helped ease my jitters about being far from home.

I wasn't sure what to expect in rehab, other than exercises to help me regain my mobility. Would it be difficult? Would it hurt? How long until I was walking again?

Shortly before I left the hospital, the traction halo was removed, so now I only had my neck collar, which supported my head, and the throat tube that cleared my lungs. I had developed a few pressure sores from staying in the same position for so long. At the time, hospitals weren't well equipped to take care of immobile patients, so I hadn't been shifted around in bed as frequently as necessary.

We were preparing to leave for Fishersville in just a couple of days: Dad would come in the plane with me, and Mom and Grandma would travel by car, meeting us there. I would miss the kind nurses I'd gotten to know at the hospital, but I was eager to jump into therapy.

The neurologist finally came to see us. This doctor was brusque and businesslike. There were no best-case scenarios or detailed explanations with him. He came in, doled out his news, and left.

"Doctor," my mother said excitedly, "we've noticed that Bryant's legs have started moving on their own. This is a good sign, right?"

"Those are just spasms," he said matter-of-factly. "Spasticity doesn't mean that he'll regain movement in his legs. Bryant has quadriplegia. His injury is incomplete, which means the spinal cord was not completely severed. But due to the level of his injury, I doubt he'll ever move more than his head again. He'll be bedridden for life and will need around-the-clock care."

Quadriplegia. Bedridden. Around-the-clock care. The words hit me like punches, each one striking a sharp blow.

Both my parents were crying. We had known my condition was serious, but until now, no one had indicated that the paralysis was permanent. We'd never expected that I, a previously active 17-year-old, on the brink of independent adulthood, would be bedridden for the rest of my life.

I didn't feel sadness or despair—I only felt anger. How dare this man come in here and so bluntly deliver such a grim diagnosis? I looked hard at that doctor with fire in in my eyes. "Doctor, I don't know what you're talking about, but you are wrong," I told him forcefully. "I *will* walk again."

I knew I would prove him wrong. The lightning strike had shown me that my life had purpose. I would do whatever it took at rehab to keep from spending the rest of my life in bed. I was going to walk again.

The lightning strike had shown me that my life had purpose. I would do whatever it took to keep from spending the rest of my life in bed.

5
a plate of french fries

On the mid-April day that my family and I left for the rehab center, we believed that I had been dealt the worst hand possible and that the road ahead of me couldn't be any harder. But I was optimistic. I had my faith and a strong support system, and I was burning with determination. Even though I knew quadriplegia meant paralysis, I was convinced that in rehab I'd get back everything I'd lost in the accident. I was entering the rehab center wheeled in on my back, but I envisioned myself walking out upright.

At Petersburg General, I was loaded onto a stretcher and driven by ambulance to the airport, where my father and I boarded a small plane to Fishersville. I was flat on my back so I couldn't see out the windows, but I asked my father, "Is the pilot bouncing off the treetops?" The small plane experienced quite a bit of turbulence, so my first plane ride was rocky.

After our short flight, my father and I rode in another ambulance to Woodrow Wilson Rehabilitation

Center. I couldn't see out the windows from my stretcher so I didn't have any first impressions of what would be my home for the next six months. I'd later learn that it was a large, rectangular brown brick building that was formerly a hospital. The interior still looked like a hospital—linoleum floors and fluorescent lights—but it didn't have a sterile hospital feel.

Once we entered and I was being wheeled down the halls to my room, I got my first look around. That short ride was eye opening. We went through a large recreation area, with a TV, tables, and chairs where patients could relax or spend time with visitors. Sitting there were several patients with physical problems like mine, but it was also clear that they no longer had the mental ability to care for themselves.

One woman in particular stood out. She was a beautiful young lady with an indentation in her forehead, right between her eyes. I later learned that she was a former Miss Virginia contestant who'd been struck by a metal pipe in a collision with a truck. The pipe flew through her windshield and in an instant her mind was destroyed.

I suddenly realized that fate had not dealt me the worst possible hand. I might not have control over my body—yet—but I had complete control of my mind. In addition to paralysis, some of these people no longer knew who or where they were. I had a much easier road ahead of me than some of these patients and their families. I never thought I'd be thankful for my condition, but my short ride had shown me an unexpected silver lining.

During my later trips around the building, I would

— ⚡ —

learn that in one corner of the rectangle was the therapy gym, with the other three corners housing different units. Unit One was for people with mental disabilities who would always need constant care, like Miss Virginia. Unit Two, where I was staying, was for those of us who had varying degrees of physical ability and who needed help caring for ourselves. Unit Three was for people who had been rehabilitated enough to learn to care for themselves. It was like a launching pad for returning to ordinary life. There was also a room for completing schoolwork or other training.

The building had originally been the Woodrow Wilson General Hospital, which primarily treated veterans from World War II. After being taken out of commission as a hospital, the building was converted by the state for use as a rehabilitation center in 1947. Back then, rehabilitation for people with disabilities was a revolutionary concept, and this was the first state-operated rehab center in the country. The doctors and staff at Woodrow Wilson were real experts in helping people with disabilities rehabilitate and get back to a productive life. I was in good hands.

When I arrived at my room, I met my new roommates: Mike, a paraplegic in his thirties; Alvin, another quadriplegic in his twenties with a cheerful disposition; and Sean, an older quadriplegic who was back in rehab after many years. He had taken some LSD that caused him to regress, mentally and physically, so he was back in rehab to regain some of his abilities. Halfway through my stay, Alvin left and a quadriplegic in his fifties named Jerry took his place. They were all friendly, convivial roommates.

We introduced ourselves, then Mike asked me, "What happened to you?"

"My pickup overturned when I swerved to miss a deer, and I broke my neck. The doctor said I'd never leave my bed, but I'm here to prove him wrong."

Each unit had a team of orderlies who were our caretakers and looked after our basic needs, as well as urology specialists and a nurse who distributed medications. In our unit, the orderlies helped with everything from getting us up and dressed in the morning to our bowel program.

Our urology needs were handled separately because of the expertise required to keep everything sterile, and in our unit urology was managed by Sally and a man named Ruesaw Sailor, who went by R.S. R.S. had been injured in the 1950s and was himself a quadriplegic, but he had regained enough control of his body that he could walk and move his arms and hands. He wore a leg brace and had a pronounced limp, but he was so manually dexterous that he could easily perform all of the complex urology tasks.

His story inspired me. When he was injured, there was so little knowledge about how to care for people with spinal cord injuries that the hospital had sent him home without so much as a catheter. "In those days, they patched you up and sent you home to die," he told me wryly.

R.S. had a great sense of humor and loved joking with us, and he always seemed to have a Coke, his favorite beverage, close at hand. He seemed to drink a case of Coke a day.

Sally was in her thirties and was cheerful, caring,

and an attentive listener. She was short with long brown hair and sparkling hazel eyes. I felt comfortable talking to her about anything and she became a close friend. She loved coffee as much as I did, and once I was able to get around in a wheelchair, I'd join her at the nurses' station for coffee—drinking mine through a straw—and a chat.

The nurse in charge of the medication cart was a feisty older lady everyone called Granny. She kept the key to the cart around her neck and I'm sure a sumo wrestler couldn't have gotten it away from her. She may have been tough, but she hadn't gotten her nickname for nothing—she was as sweet and caring as a grandmother. We saw the doctor so infrequently that I can't even recall his name, but the urologists, orderlies, nurses, and therapists felt as close as family.

My mother and Grandma Neville had traveled to Fishersville separately and were boarding in a private home in Waynesboro so they could visit me each day. Seeing them kept my spirits up and gave me something to look forward to. Grandma was a social butterfly and wasted no time getting to know the other patients. She'd spend part of each day visiting others, especially those whose families were far away and couldn't visit. Mom and I loved watching Grandma make her rounds.

My father stayed in DeWitt to continue working, but he visited us many weekends. Dad's sister Nancy and her husband, George, often visited him and our Chihuahua, Penny, keeping them company and helping around the house during the months Mom and Grandma were with me. I knew it was difficult for my family to be separated and was grateful to see them so often, as some patients never had visitors.

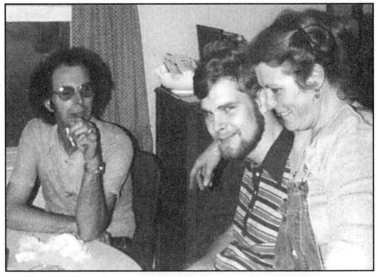

R.S. and Sally took care of my unit's urology needs. R.S. had overcome paralysis and inspired me. Sally became a dear friend and confidante.

I was chomping at the bit to jump into therapy when I first arrived, but the staff told me, "Not so fast." There were medical issues to address first. I had a bladder infection and low fever that hadn't been properly treated at the hospital, so Granny gave me some injections of a powerful antibiotic that cleared it up. Then my tracheotomy tube was removed so that the hole in my throat could close and I could spend a few days strengthening my breathing abilities.

Before my pressure sores could be treated, I had to be able to sit up. I assumed someone would prop me upright in a chair and I'd be on my way. The reality was more complicated. The first two or three days, a therapist named Mary Beth raised the back of the bed a bit so I was propped at an angle, but that was it. I was frustrated. I hadn't sat upright in a month and was eager to try it.

When she finally swung my legs off the side of the bed and sat me upright, everything went black.

I came to after a few moments, lying back in the bed. The experience was disturbingly similar to when my heart stopped at the hospital.

"What happened?"

"You lost consciousness," said Mary Beth. "You've been lying flat for so long your body has forgotten how to regulate your blood pressure. We'll ease you back into remembering. Let's try it again."

Once again, I was propped up and my legs were swung over the side of the bed. Once again, I blacked out for a few seconds. This was repeated over and over until I could be propped up in bed with my legs over the side. Then we moved on to getting me upright in a wheelchair. When I'd black out in the wheelchair, Mary Beth would tilt the chair back on its rear wheels until I came to. My body felt heavy, like I weighed a thousand pounds.

It took about a week until I regained enough strength to sit upright in the wheelchair. I wasn't yet strong enough to hold my head upright so I still had on a neck collar for support. Instead of shoes I wore soft sheepskin booties that protected my feet from rubbing against each other and forming more sores. Even wearing shoes, I learned, was something I'd have to gradually work my way up to doing. If just sitting was this hard, I couldn't imagine what physical therapy would bring.

When I could sit without passing out, I began therapy. The hospital hadn't been equipped to care for my pressure sores, but at Woodrow Wilson they had whirlpool treatments, special dressings and medicines, and the expertise to educate me on caring for my skin.

I learned how to shift in my wheelchair to avoid developing further sores. I also started using a ROHO cushion, a special inflatable pillow with adjustable nodules that constantly shifted the pressure of my seated body, helping me avoid the formation of new sores.

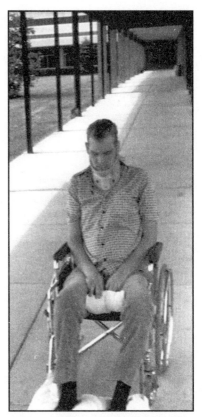

Half of my days were spent in physical therapy and half in occupational therapy. Physical therapy helped me develop and exercise my muscles so my arms and legs would remain limber. The therapy room was full of mats, weights, exercise equipment, and a whirlpool. Occupational therapy built on physical therapy to help me relearn

At Woodrow Wilson Rehabilitation Center, it took me days just to learn to sit. This was taken shortly after I was able to sit upright—I could only stay seated for short periods of time.

basic skills like using utensils. The occupational therapy room looked like a house without walls, with different areas set up like a kitchen, a bedroom, and a living room.

Andrea, or Andy, was my physical therapist. When I first met her I was sure she wouldn't be able to move me without help because she was so petite and I was at least a foot taller. Yet the first time she picked me up, she did it gracefully without so much as a grunt. She was tough, and her philosophy was "No pain, no gain."

Because my spinal cord break was in the third through fifth vertebrae, I couldn't move my arms and hands freely like a paraplegic, but there was a chance of regaining some mobility in my upper arms. We started with stretching my stiff limbs, a painful exercise after a month of lying still.

Despite my paralysis, I could still feel some sensations in my limbs, similar to the pins-and-needles feeling that happens when one's arm or foot falls asleep. The worst stretch was when Andy put my legs straight out in front of me then pulled my arms behind me, as if I were sitting on them. Yow, that hurt! But these painful stretches were necessary to keep me limber and prevent atrophying and tightening in my limbs.

I couldn't move anything other than my head and shoulders. Andy wanted to see if we could get any movement from my arms. She asked me to concentrate and try to move my arm. I focused very hard and after several days of trying we saw a small twinge in my left arm.

"That's good, Bryant!"

The discouraging words I'd heard from the neurologist at the hospital haunted me.

"Are you sure it's not just a spasm?" I asked.

"Try to do it again."

I tried. Another twinge!

Andy beamed. "Looks to me like that was all you making that movement. That was conscious movement—not a spasm."

"So this is a good sign?"

"I'll say! Let's keep going." I was relieved and proud. I had made my arm move!

As we worked to explore my abilities, I learned that I could move my biceps but not my triceps, meaning I could make pulling motions but not pushing ones. Soon Andy strapped small weights to my arms—which felt enormous—to help build the muscles and increase my range of motion.

Every day I could move a tiny bit more. Soon I could prop my elbow on the table and lift my hand slightly off the surface. We kept at this, trying it over and over again, until I could raise my hand higher and higher. Much of therapy was repetitive and slow going, but the excitement over every incremental improvement kept me motivated. I would show that doctor. It had only been a few weeks since I'd left the hospital and I was already disproving his diagnosis of "bedridden for life."

At first, because I was relearning how to move, occupational therapy was an extension of physical therapy. But once I began moving my arms, occupational therapy focused on things like writing my name or eating. Mary Beth was my occupational therapist and Andy's physical opposite. She was my height and solidly built. Once I was able to raise my left hand off the table, Mary Beth said, "Okay, let's see if we can get you using a fork."

I looked at her with a raised eyebrow. "I can't move my fingers. How can I do that?"

"We're prepared for all kinds of situations here," she said. "We've got special straps and attachments that will help you swing your arm over to your mouth."

She set up a contraption of metal rods on my chair that had a sling where I could rest my elbow and take the weight off my arm. "Now, try bringing your hand to your face." Once I'd mastered this movement, she added a white felt strap to my hand that held a fork. "Now try to bring the fork to your mouth."

I had to be careful to avoid stabbing myself, but in time I was able to successfully bring the fork to my mouth.

"Great!" Mary Beth chirped. "Now let's have some real fun and see what you can do." She produced a plate of French fries, which I loved—the perfect motivator.

I thought setting a plate of one of my favorite foods in front of me that I couldn't get to was no fair! But Mary Beth was tough. There was no cheating. If I couldn't get the French fry myself, I wouldn't get one. Period.

For two hours I tried to get just one fry on my fork. The fry would slip off the fork or I'd knock it off the plate, but I kept trying. Those darned French fries made me work harder than ever. Mary Beth was smart—I doubt I'd have made such an effort if they'd been green beans.

Finally, after a couple of days I managed to slip the fork securely under a fry, a major breakthrough. Now all I had to do was get it to my mouth. I started to raise the fork. The fry remained balanced on it. My mouth watered in anticipation. I might actually make this.

But halfway to my mouth, the fry fell off the fork. I could have cried, I was so deflated. But Mary Beth was enthusiastic. "Now you can say you've gotten the food halfway to your mouth!" She and the rest of the staff always saw the glass as half full.

By the end of that day, I managed to get a fry all the way to my mouth. It was cold and stale but was the most delicious French fry I'd ever eaten. I chewed blissfully and beamed at Mary Beth.

Cold and stale, it was the most delicious French fry I'd ever eaten.

She smiled and nodded. "I'll give you one thing, you sure are determined!"

After several more days of fork work, I could control my movements enough to feed myself for the first time since the accident. With the exception of breakfast, which was fed to us in bed, I was expected to feed myself during lunch and dinner. This small degree of personal independence was a monumental victory for me. Now I could eat most foods with my fork, as long as my meal was cut into small pieces for me. Using a spoon was much harder, but I figured out how to eat things like soup without one. I used the fork to eat the pieces of food in the bowl, then I drank the broth with a straw. I was a teenager with a seemingly endless appetite, so when it came to food, I was highly motivated to figure out how to eat it!

After a couple of months, I was strong enough to lift my elbow and control my arm without the support sling, so I only needed the hand strap to use my fork. I also learned to write with another special hand strap, and I went from being a righty to a lefty because my left arm was stronger. My handwriting style had changed, but I was fiercely proud that I could sign my name and write short notes.

I was glad Mom and Grandma came to visit every afternoon, but I missed seeing Dad. I knew that with my mother unemployed, our family needed the income and health insurance Dad's job provided. I enjoyed showing him my progress during his weekend visits.

Other friends and family visited too, with the notable exception of my great-aunt Kathleen, whom we called Steen. There had been a sisterly feud between her and Grandma Neville and they were avoiding each other. Steen also suffered from arthritis and spent a lot of time in bed. I missed her and her husband, Peter (or Pa), so one day I phoned her.

She sounded weak. "Hey, Bryant. How you doing?"

"I'm doing all right, Steen, but I'd be a lot better if I could see you and Pa. I miss you both so much."

"We miss you too."

"I hope I get to see you both soon. It would make me feel so much better. I miss playing cards with you."

Maybe I got lucky, or maybe I had challenged Steen to get out of bed. Either way, the following week, Steen and Pa drove up to Fishersville in their camper, set themselves up at a nearby campground, and except for a few weekends when they traveled home, visited me every day.

This led to another wonderful thing—Steen and Grandma made up. It was a comfort to see something good come out of my accident. I had managed to get over the blame and the anger, and I was working hard to make the best of things and understand my life's new direction. But the thing I felt best about was seeing Steen out of bed and reconciled with her sister. Until the day she died, Steen never again let her arthritis defeat her and instead stayed positive and as active as possible.

School was in session and my friends were busy, but they visited whenever they could on weekends. Visits from Amy were always a big treat. I eagerly showed off my latest accomplishments from therapy. She would smile and say, "That's great, Bryant! I'm so happy for you." It made me feel so warm inside when she would praise me.

It was a comfort to see something good come out of my accident. I had managed to get over the blame and the anger.

Amy remained loyal to me and despite the physical distance I felt closer to her than ever. Every Wednesday, and on weekends when she didn't visit, someone would help me dial her number from a pay phone in the hall that was specially designed to hold the receiver for those of us in wheelchairs. She'd catch me up on news about our classmates and I'd share what was going on at the center. And we shared lots of exciting plans for my eventual return home: weekends together, attending the senior prom, graduation.

Amy's loving support helped me face the harder days in rehab. She cheered me on when I succeeded and encouraged me when I was frustrated. I couldn't imagine life back home without her. She was undaunted by the challenges I faced, and I felt lucky to have her by my side.

In June, I started visiting home on weekends, leaving Fishersville with Mom and Grandma on Friday afternoon and returning Sunday afternoon. My parents, primarily my mother, were learning the skills and purchasing the equipment needed to help me with my urology and bowel needs as well as helping me in and out of my wheelchair. They were endlessly patient and positive, just as eager as I was to learn how to adapt to my new life.

It became clear during my weekend visits that other changes were necessary to accommodate me. Sitting in the cramped car for the four-hour ride was difficult—I would have been more comfortable lying flat or staying in my wheelchair. The family house had only one floor, but it was still challenging to navigate certain spots in my wheelchair, especially my bedroom. These changes required money, and my parents' finances were already stretched.

When our community learned what had happened to me and how my family needed help to modify our home and car, friends and strangers alike rallied in support. Friends and family at the Rocky Run Methodist Church, Bott Memorial Presbyterian Church, and Hawkins Memorial Presbyterian Church organized a fundraising walk-a-thon. The local Moose Lodge held an auction, and other community groups played a charity softball game and organized fundraising dinners. I was deeply touched and made it a point to go home for the walk-a-thon on June 27.

There were signs welcoming me home and balloons everywhere. Over one hundred walkers staggered their start times and walked a six-mile stretch of country roads, ending at my house, so I got to see a steady stream of well-wishers all day. After a crowd had gathered in our yard, W. C. Knott, the county administrator, read everyone an inspiring letter written to me by President Ronald Reagan. Someone had managed to get him information about my story and he had sent me a letter, enclosing an autographed photo.

"Mrs. Reagan and I are only two of a great number of people who care about you," President Reagan wrote to me. "There is a divine plan for all us. It seems that part of yours is to generate much love and caring from others. Today you are surrounded by your friends and neighbors from DeWitt in a spirit of fellowship and goodwill, and it must be a source of strength to know that you have inspired so many people."

Later that night, I was driven to my Uncle Tom's house, where he hosted a fundraising stew dinner for me, sponsored by the Darvills Ruritan Club and my dad's plant. It was a long, exhausting day but it was gratifying to see that so many people supported me and my family. I felt like a minor celebrity.

My father had gotten a loan from the local Bank of McKenney to purchase a van and modify it for my needs. The bank president didn't charge interest, and the walk-a-thon funds paid back the loan.

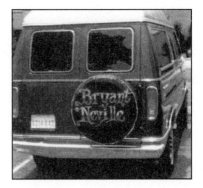

At the end of the walk, the organizers presented me with the specially equipped blue Ford van. The front seats were intact, but the back rows had been removed to fit my wheelchair. The top of the van had been lifted to accommodate my height. It had a lift, as well as straps for holding the wheelchair in place. It also had a bed, so I could ride lying down on longer trips. The spare tire cover on the back of the van had my name on it in fancy script.

The other fundraisers helped my family renovate the house to accommodate my wheelchair and personal needs. Dad has some contractor friends who completed all the renovations to our home free of charge—he only had to purchase the materials. They built a new, larger bedroom, complete with a modified bathroom, and an attached, covered carport for getting my wheelchair in and out of the house with ease.

Every time I rode to or from Fishersville in the van, I remembered that my parents and I weren't in this alone. The outpouring of support from loved ones and strangers alike kept me working as hard as I could to regain my strength and skills in rehab and kept my spirits high.

With so much positive energy around me, I couldn't possibly fail.

DeWitt Residents Rally To Help Paralyzed Youth

By KENT BOOTH
Progress-Index Staff Writer

DeWITT — Bryant Neville was driving home from a date shortly after midnight March 21 when, a mile from his home, he spotted a deer in the road.

The 17-year-old DeWitt youth slowed down and started pulling his small pick-up truck over to the side of the road. But, for some unknown reason, a tire caught on the soft shoulder of the road and the truck flipped over onto its roof.

Bryant — an active young man and honor roll student — was paralyzed from the neck down.

"I was laying there for 30 minutes before someone finally came by," he recalled recently, "but it seemed like about 20 hours. I was never unconscious but I couldn't feel anything. All I could do was move my head."

Bryant is currently undergoing physical and occupational therapy at the Woodrow Wilson Rehabilitation Center in Fishersville. But his friends haven't forgotten about him.

Saturday morning Bryant's friends, former classmates and supporters walked 12 miles to raise money to help with his family's medical expenses and other bills. The walk-a-thon, which was sponsored by the nearby Rocky Run Methodist Church, included a stop at Bryant's home on State Route 645.

Bryant broke his fifth and sixth vertebrae, which are in the neck area, and severed his spinal cord. But his medical problems didn't end there.

After undergoing an operation at Petersburg General Hospital, in which a piece of his hip bone was surgically removed and fused with his neck to strengthen it, Bryant came down with pneumonia. And he twice suffered heart failure while at PGH.

Bryant spent four weeks at PGH — 3½ of which were spent in the intensive care unit. Then, on April 22, he was flown to the rehabilitation center in Fishersville.

The popular youth, whose home is overrun by friends every time he comes back to visit, is slowly regaining some movement.

"I can move my left arm pretty good, and I'm getting to where I can also move my right arm," he said in a telephone interview last week. "But I don't have any use in my fingers yet ... I've been going along pretty fast in the rehabilitation up here but it seems slow to me. It's a big change."

A junior last year at Dinwiddie County Senior High School, Bryant was an honor roll student and a member of the Future Farmers of America. The tall, blonde-haired youth enjoyed hunting, fishing, golf and baseball.

Bryant's confidence in himself has never waned.

"I'm just confident I'm going to get it all (movement) back; I don't know how long it'll take," he said.

His parents can attest to the positive outlook and determination.

"It's unbelievable how he's handled it ... I would have given up," noted his mother, Mrs. Gloria Neville. "Each time he comes back more determined than ever."

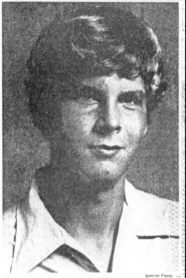

Bryant Neville Is Determined To Recover
This is a high school picture taken before accident.

Mrs. Neville, who taught second grade at Southside Elementary School before the accident, is staying at the hospital with Bryant. She rents a room in nearby Waynesboro.

"Bryant has a real strong faith," said his father, James B. Neville Sr., who is superintendent of the Continental Forest Industries plant in McKenney. "He's just got the attitude that he's going to lick this thing."

Bryant, who is an only child, had been home three times before this weekend. He travels back and forth in a custom-built 1979 Ford van which his family purchased.

Due to Bryant's height — he is six feet, three inches tall — the Nevilles had to have the roof raised 12 inches. Mr. Neville and his brother, who lives next door, are in the process of installing a wheelchair lift in the van.

Bryant's father is also planning to install ramps around the house and remodel the youth's bedroom and bathroom to accommodate his situation.

Bryant, who will return to the rehabilitation center around 4:30 this afternoon, will probably be there for anywhere from three to five months. Meanwhile, he is busy regaining his strength.

"You stay busy," he said about the rehabilitation program. "From 8 (o'clock) to 4, it's work ... It takes a whole lot out of you but it's worth it."

6
tough love

From the first time I'd heard the doctor say words like "quadriplegia" and "paralysis," I'd never stopped believing that my condition was temporary. I'd envisioned myself slowly but surely regaining the use of my arms and legs and walking out of rehab, just like R.S.

After months of slow, hard work in therapy, I began accepting that I would never walk again. R.S. still inspired me, but I realized that his ability to regain the use of his legs was an exception, not the rule. Woodrow Wilson's staff supported all patients in coming to grips with their conditions on their own terms and in their own time. I never once heard anyone use phrases like "you will never" or "you cannot," and no one ever pushed me to accept that my paralysis was permanent.

Instead, our care focused on encouraging us to adapt to our new reality and finding ways to live in the aftermath of our injuries. My legs still twitched sometimes, but this was solely due to spasticity—I couldn't consciously cause them to move. After weeks of therapy and reflection, I accepted that I'd now live on four wheels instead of two feet.

It was difficult knowing that I'd never again play baseball, drive my car, or even pour my own cup of coffee, but I didn't let these limitations defeat me and instead was grateful for what I could still do. I had complete control over my mind, unlike some of my fellow patients. And unlike some quadriplegics, I had regained some arm movement, allowing me to use utensils and pens. Knowing that the alternative to a wheelchair was being bedridden, I gladly took the wheelchair.

In addition to learning new ways of using my body, I also learned to rely on others for help with tasks I'd previously taken for granted. Getting out of bed and dressed, getting around, and performing personal hygiene—from brushing my teeth to emptying my bowels—all required help. I quickly learned to overcome my modesty, be patient, and keep a good sense of humor. Staying positive and laughing at myself kept me from being embarrassed.

My personal needs were now on a schedule. Some of the more able-bodied patients, like the paraplegics, were able to handle their catheters and bowel programs by themselves. But as a quadriplegic, I was permanently dependent on others for these important tasks. Now there were six scheduled times a day, once every four hours, when my bladder was emptied using a catheter.

The previously insignificant act of peeing now took about ten minutes. Sticking to such a strict regimen seemed annoying but was important. Failure to empty a full bladder can cause a condition called autonomic dysreflexia—a life-threatening overstimulation of the nervous system resulting in a very high jump in blood pressure, severe throbbing headache, profuse sweating and flushed skin, and extreme anxiety. If this was left untreated, it could lead to a stroke. I unfortunately experienced this a few times and the sharp pains in my head felt like I was being hit with an axe. My family and I quickly learned how important it was to stick to the schedule.

Bowel movements were on a schedule too, and many of the men in my unit were on the same twice-a-week regimen. A couple of suppositories were inserted and then we sat on commodes in the bathroom waiting to go. Two rooms of four men each adjoined each bathroom, so every Monday and Thursday there were eight of us sitting in the bathroom together, naked on potty chairs waiting to poop.

I'd never imagined scheduled bowel movements, let alone doing something so private among company! I knew there was no other way around it, so I just chuckled and took it in stride. At least there were others in the same boat!

Knowing that my family would care for me at home kept my spirits high. Some patients never had visitors and had little or no outside support. Another quadriplegic named Kevin, whose upper body was less mobile than mine, inspired and impressed me. His family wasn't involved in his life, and after rehab he would move to a nursing home with constant care—yet he was always smiling and laughing. Knowing he faced such adversity with a smile made me all the more grateful to have a strong support system.

On the opposite end of the spectrum, there were some patients who thought their situation was the worst imaginable. My roommate Mike would sometimes fall into a funk of self-pity. One morning he asked R.S., "Can you help me get out of bed?"

Mike was a paraplegic and could use his upper body to get out of bed and into his

I'd never imagined scheduled bowel movements, let alone doing something so private among company!

wheelchair, so I thought this was an unusual request, but R.S. just said, "Okay." He limped over to Mike's bed, grabbed him by his chest hair, and yanked him upright.

"Ow! What'd you do that for?" Mike growled, rubbing his chest.

R.S. just chuckled. "Tough love," he said.

Mike never again asked for help getting out of bed. He realized he was fortunate to have more independence than many of us—as well as fearing the loss of more chest hair. The folks at the center, R.S. included, were some of the most compassionate people I'd met, but they also knew compassion could mean pushing a person out of his comfort zone. Whether it was my therapist Andy urging me to lift a weight a few more times or R.S. showing Mike he could get up alone, these people knew tough love kept us from giving up on ourselves.

The first wheelchair I used at the center was manual. Sometimes I had to wait to be fetched, and other times I was left stranded mid-trip because the person pushing me had to attend to something more urgent. I just reminded myself to be patient—I'd get where I needed to go eventually, and there were usually people around to chat with while I waited. After I built up my arm muscles, I was able to navigate short distances using push knobs on the wheels, but I still relied on being pushed longer distances.

It wasn't until later in the summer that I tried an electric wheelchair, which I operated by pushing a joystick. I was still learning to use my arms so my navigation wasn't always accurate and I ran into things. A few times, I had a leg spasm, which threw me off kilter in the seat, and I'd have to wait for someone to reseat me properly.

Once when I had a spasm, I tried to hold myself upright using the joystick but instead slumped over with my hand pressed against it. I found myself turning round and round in circles in the middle of the hall, hoping someone would help before I fell dizzily out of the seat.

Another time as I was driving along, my hand slipped off the joystick. The chairs weren't designed to stop on a dime, but they came pretty close. The next thing I knew, I was dumped in a heap on the floor, staring back at the chair through my legs, hollering, "Help!" Riding it wasn't foolproof, but I loved getting around the building on my own. Soon I could drive to the nurses' station for regular coffee breaks with Sally. She was quite proud of my progress.

I planned to return to my high school and finish senior year with my classmates, so I completed the junior year assignments on my own between therapy sessions. The year was nearly over so it wasn't too difficult to get caught up. When I applied myself to my studies, the work wasn't that hard. My grades had slipped because I'd been distracted and lacked motivation.

I tried to hold myself upright using the joystick and found myself turning round and round in circles.

Big Daddy used to say, "Use your head for something other than a hat rack," and now I took his words to heart. The tree that had been blasted to bits by lightning was my sign that my life had a purpose. To fulfill that purpose, I'd have to learn skills that were mental rather than physical, which meant going to college. I vowed to work hard my senior year to get good grades.

During the summer I continued traveling home most weekends. The van made the trip comfortable, and spending time with my friends and Amy kept my spirits high. I also enjoyed seeing the improvements made to our home that would help me get around. The weekends home were trial runs for my parents, who practiced their skills in caring for me.

There was certainly a learning curve for all of us. One evening I had a leg spasm while lying in bed. The force jerked me over the edge, and on my way to the floor I wacked my head on each shelf of the bookshelf next to my bed. I wasn't terribly hurt, but this taught my parents and me two important lessons: make sure I was centered in the bed away from the edge, and give the bed a wide berth. As we all grew accustomed to my situation and needs, the awkward moments were fewer and further between.

—— ⚡ ——

My relationship with Amy continued to grow stronger and more serious. She knew my disability brought with it unique challenges, and yet her love didn't falter. I felt confident that she was the one. Maybe we would even get married someday. I hoped so, because I didn't want to give up on my lifelong dream of having a family. I knew she wanted a family too, so we seemed fated to stay together.

One weekend in July, Amy let me know that her parents would be out of town and she'd have the house to herself. Even though we had been together for a while before the accident, we hadn't yet had sex, so we planned to have our first time together that weekend. It was important to us to share this meaningful experience, but my size made it nearly impossible for her to lift me out of my chair and into bed. My cousin Johnny came to the rescue. I could trust him to be discreet, so he picked me up at my parents' home, drove me to Amy's, and helped me lie in bed before leaving us alone.

It was a very tender moment, but physically things didn't go as planned. I loved Amy and wanted her so much, but I couldn't get aroused. I was frustrated and embarrassed, and she seemed to be too.

"Don't worry," she brushed it off, but she seemed troubled.

I should have pushed her to discuss what was truly bothering her and voiced my own concerns, but instead we both ignored it. I spent the next few days pondering what had happened—or hadn't happened. Was there something wrong with me? Was this just a fluke, or was this the way it would always be? I worried that I could no longer have sex normally, and this thought was so dispiriting and scary that I tried desperately to push it out of my mind.

Once I was back at the center, I was anxious about my Wednesday call with Amy. Would she bring up our botched weekend? Would I? Or would we once again ignore my failure in bed? When I called her, she seemed distant and subdued, unlike her usual happy self.

I already suspected the answer but couldn't help asking, "What's wrong?"

"Oh, nothing."

But I knew it wasn't nothing. Now I was sure that weekend's events had upset her. Sticking our heads in the sand hadn't helped so I pressed further until she finally relented.

"Bryant, I've been thinking a lot about what you said to me, back at the hospital when you were first hurt, and I think you were right. I don't think that we should stay together after all."

I'd never expected this. It felt like I was back in the truck, trapped upside down and unable to take a breath. I struggled to regain myself. "What? Why?"

"I think we're on different paths. I just don't think we should stay together, is all," she said softly.

The conversation continued for a few more awkward minutes, but my brain was reeling so I stopped listening. Finally we said goodbye and hung up. I sat next to the phone, stunned and numb. I couldn't believe Amy had broken up with me. I knew things hadn't gone as planned, but how could she leave me? We'd been through so much together—the times when I nearly died in the hospital, the long stretches of time apart from each other, the realization that I would never walk again. She'd had

— ⚡ —

many opportunities to leave me before and hadn't, so it had to be because I'd failed at sex.

I plunged into depths so low I felt like I'd never surface again. If I couldn't have sex with a woman I loved, what kind of a man was I? How would I ever fulfill my dream of getting married and starting a family? What if I never had the chance to be a lover, husband, and father?

I felt like the biblical character Job, who had one misfortune after another heaped on him, but now I was at my breaking point. I had lived through the accident, the near-death experiences at the hospital, the pressure sores, and the pneumonia; I had to abandon my modesty and depend on others for every personal need; I had to relearn how to use my body in limited ways; I would never walk again.

It had been a difficult few months, but I had worked hard to overcome each challenge, adapting to my radically new life and keeping a positive attitude. None of these things had defeated me. Now I had been robbed of my manhood. The indignity and sorrow crushed me. What was left for me if I couldn't even feel like a whole man?

This was the lowest point in my life—not Big Daddy's death, not the accident, not the knowledge that I'd never walk again. It was that phone call with Amy. I hated her for bringing me to this level of despair and wished I had the ability to kill myself, because ending my life felt like the best option.

I didn't want to talk to anybody, putting on a brave face for my family and friends so they wouldn't suspect something was wrong. My parents didn't know what had happened between Amy and me—we were a close family, but discussing my sex life as a 17-year-old with my mother or father seemed terribly taboo, so I kept my mouth shut.

If I couldn't have sex with a woman I loved, what kind of a man was I? How would I ever fulfill my dream?

The staff knew me well enough to realize something was wrong. R.S. especially tried to draw it out of me, but it was Sally who finally got me to open up. Her persistent yet gentle coaxing persuaded me to confide in her. Talking to a woman about sex was the last thing I'd ever considered, but I knew I could trust her.

As we sat together talking privately, I told her what had happened, stumbling over my words in embarrassment. "My girlfriend and I were together, and we were trying to—you know—take it to the next level." I felt myself flushing, but Sally's concerned look urged me on. "And when we tried to… be together, nothing happened for me. A few days later she decided she didn't want to stay with me, and I know it's because I couldn't perform, and now I don't know what to do." I pushed on. "I hate knowing that I'm not a man—not really, not in that way. What's the point of anything?"

Sally nodded knowingly. "Bryant, I know you must be worried that you will never have a normal sex life. But since you have an incomplete spinal cord injury, you are still physically able to have sex. Some people's spinal cord injuries cause impotence, but yours does not."

I must have looked confused. "But if I still can, why

didn't anything happen that night?"

"Because now, instead of being mentally aroused, your body must be physically aroused to have an erection. Things still work—they just work in a different way. Think about when someone is inserting your catheter. You often get erections then, and it's certainly not because you're mentally aroused—it's all physical."

I couldn't believe how openly she was discussing all of this, without a trace of embarrassment. "So as long as someone touches me, I would still be able to...?"

Sally smiled. "Yes. You just have to adapt to this new way of doing things. There are some videos and books here that explain things further. I'll get them for you. Any time you have questions or you want to know more about something, you just come to me."

A wave of relief washed over me. "I wish someone had told me this stuff before," I said. "It's so hard to talk about."

"But it's important," she replied. "You have to do a lot of things differently in your life now, but just because you've got a disability doesn't mean you can't feel like a whole person. Sex is important."

"You don't know how much this means to me," I told her. "Thank you so much for this. I feel like I'm getting my life back."

"Anything I can do to help. I hate seeing you so miserable. Will you stop moping around now?"

"Yes," I told her.

My talk with Sally lifted me out of my depression. Even though I was paralyzed, I was still a man. Now I knew what had happened—or not happened—wasn't my fault or Amy's. I thought about calling her and trying to discuss things with her now that I was educated, but she'd made it clear that she wanted to us to go our separate ways, so I didn't.

"So as long as someone touches me, I would still be able to...?" Sally smiled. "Yes."

I was able to start healing the anger I felt toward Amy. I realized that she didn't want to take the chance of not fulfilling her dreams of motherhood. Months earlier in the hospital, I had tried to convince her to do exactly what she had done now and leave me. Now I could see that she had every right to get what she desired from life. Our breakup still hurt me, but at least I was able to release the hatred and anger.

I turned to Sally often as a resource with many questions and concerns. The books and videos helped, but it was hearing things from her that truly reassured me. She never made me feel foolish or embarrassed. No one had ever been so honest and open with me about something as sensitive as sex. I felt like I owed my life to her—I'm certain I would have stayed terribly depressed if she hadn't convinced me to confide in her.

The mind of a 17-year-old boy on the rebound is a dangerous place, and at this point, I imagined what Sally and I had surpassed friendship. She was my dearest friend and confidante and I couldn't imagine spending my life with anyone else. She was at least 15 years my senior, but I was certain she was the woman for me. I'd transferred my romantic feelings for Amy and now Sally was the one. My goal to make something of my life was now grounded in impressing her. I knew she cared deeply for me so I made my intentions clear.

"Just wait, Sally," I'd say. "I'm going to do something really great, and then I'll come back for you and we'll be together."

She always just laughed. "You just focus on getting well and back to life and then we'll see what happens." She was never dismissive, but she also never actually agreed to my plan. This didn't faze me. I was certain that when she saw how successful I became, she'd have no qualms about being with me.

By October, the doctor determined that I'd regained enough strength and mobility in my arms to return home. As my discharge day approached, I felt a mixture of sadness and excitement. I would miss the staff, who felt like a second family, and I was anxious about leaving the safety of the center's routines. But I missed my friends and relatives and couldn't wait to return home and go back to school, where I was determined to excel.

The day arrived, and as my parents gathered my belongings and prepared the van for the drive home, I said my goodbyes. There were lots of laughs, a few tears, and requests to keep in touch and come back to visit. It was hardest to say goodbye to Sally. She hugged me tightly. "Remember to write, okay?"

I looked back at her intently, love and determination burning in my eyes. "Of course. I'll be back, Sally."

My parents got me settled into the van and we drove back to DeWitt. I was ready for the next chapter of my life.

7
more than a hatrack

It was great to be back home with my parents and near my friends and relatives. My new room was comfortable and it was easy to get around the renovated house. As my parents and I adjusted to our new routines, I stayed positive and patient. I knew we were all doing our best, and I was grateful that my parents uncomplainingly cared for me, so I didn't mind if things took longer to do or went awry sometimes. Our relatives helped us too and visited often. Steen and Pa still came over regularly to play cards with us, with me using a special card holder, and both my grandmothers still loved to dote on me.

I decided to use a manual wheelchair at home. Using the push knobs to move short distances would help keep my arms strong, and my friends and family were eager to push me longer distances. It was comforting to always have a companion by my side to help.

It was mid-October, and I couldn't wait to see my classmates and start my classes.

—⚡—

I was determined to get back to straight A's so I could go to college. Now that my future livelihood depended on my mental skills, I'd need an advanced degree so I could get a good job, contribute to my household, and lead a productive life.

The only thing I worried about was seeing Amy. How would we act around each other? Would it be awkward or painful? I had let go of much of my anger over our breakup but was still concerned. I reminded myself that Amy was now part of my past; Sally was my future, so I would focus on her and not let my failed relationship upset me.

Being dependent on my parents for my care meant sticking to a daily routine. Each morning my parents would get me out of bed, dressed, and in my wheelchair for breakfast. Then my mother would help me wash my face, shave, and brush my teeth.

Jimmy Stidham would be driving me to and from school each day in my van, but my mother was concerned about who would help with my catheter. I needed to empty my bladder every four hours, and one of those times was during the school day. She explained that the school was figuring out if a nurse could come in to do it when Jimmy piped up.

"I can do it," he offered. "Just show me what I need to do."

Mom was relieved—she knew she could trust Jimmy. She showed him how to use the catheter kit and made sure he always had a supply available. The kits are sealed, sterile bags containing a thin 16-inch-long tube, three betadine sterilization swabs, and a package of lubrication. First the swabs were wiped over the urethral opening in my penis, then the tube was lubricated and inserted until it entered my bladder. This allowed the urine to flow into the collection bag. Jimmy may not have known the term autonomic dysreflexia, but he did know that if I didn't empty my bladder on schedule, I could get very sick and even die. He took his responsibility very seriously.

> Whatever the future held, I didn't see any harm in having a little romance in the meantime.

Every day at lunchtime, we went to the teachers' lounge so Jimmy could cath me. I'd gotten over my modesty issues at rehab, so the fact that the teachers were witnessing a private bodily function didn't bother me. Seeing our teachers socializing together outside the classroom, talking about their lives just like any other adults, made me realize they were not some alien species!

Since my car and spending money were gone, fewer acquaintances joined me at the bowling alley and pool hall. But my close friends—Jimmy, Jamie, and Walter— were loyal and always included me in plans. They treated me like the same old Bryant, not a guy in a wheelchair. I learned that it was better to have a few close friends than to be popular.

I even went on dates with a few girls. Thanks to Sally's advice, I knew I could still have a love life. Part of me still believed that someday I'd be with her, but as the weeks passed, my time at Woodrow Wilson was becoming part of my past and my infatuation diminished. Whatever the future held, I didn't see any harm in having a little romance in the meantime. None of the dates led to anything serious, but it was still fun to go out and flirt. Because the girls always agreed to go out with me, my confidence soared—until I asked a girl to the senior prom.

"Bryant, I'd love to go with you, but I need to check if it's okay with my boyfriend."

Ouch! These girls had been going out with me because they felt bad saying no! I had been convinced that I was still popular and attractive, but this comment completely deflated my ego. I managed to sputter, "Don't sweat it. Sorry to have bothered you!" and retreated with my tail between my legs. It was a bitter, painful pill to swallow, but at that point I decided to turn my attention solely to my studies. No more dances, no more dates. I'd shelf romance for now and instead focus on getting into college and finding a good career.

Another blow to my romantic ego came when I learned that Amy and my cousin Steve started dating. I couldn't believe it—was she using him as a substitute for me? We looked similar and our personalities were somewhat similar too, and for a while I jealously seethed that she was just reliving our relationship with an able-bodied version of me. This wasn't fair to either of them, but the wounds from our breakup were still fresh. Even though I'd resolved to focus on my studies and forget about Amy, it still hurt. Maybe I should have confided in Steve how much it bothered me, but I felt I couldn't say anything because he had saved my life the night of the accident. I tried to ignore their relationship and was secretly relieved that it was short-lived.

Focusing intently on my coursework helped me

rediscover my love of learning. I enjoyed and did well in every class, but attending school in a wheelchair presented some challenges. I was no longer able to take extensive notes, but I had a great memory and could remember the lecture material without having to write much down. When it came to taking tests, the teachers would usually sit next to me and write down the answers I dictated. And since this was before the Americans with Disabilities Act passed, the school was not required to provide ramps and elevators. There were some stairs I had to contend with, but my friends grabbed onto my chair and lifted me where I needed to go.

That year, the school got its first computer, a TRS-80 Tandy, which was kept in the library. I was intrigued and determined to figure out how to use it. During my study hall period, I fooled around with it, with a friend typing for me, and soon I mastered one of the computer languages and was even able to write programs. We ordered a special arm strap from Woodrow Wilson that was designed to hold a pencil with a large eraser. By moving my arm over the keyboard, I could use the eraser end of the pencil to type unassisted.

The computer was endlessly fascinating and I loved using it. Here was something I was good at that I could easily work on independently. It was still the early days of personal computing, but I could see the advantage to learning about these machines. As I considered colleges, I made sure to look for one that had computer classes.

During my senior year, I made a special new friend. That year, a woman named Etta Rossman became the first female pastor to take over at my father's original church, Hawkins Memorial Presbyterian Church. Most of Dad's siblings and Grandma Neville still attended Hawkins Church and got to know Reverend Rossman well. Many of the churchgoers were initially apprehensive about having a woman pastor, but her inspirational, captivating sermons and gracious, caring demeanor soon won them over and she was welcomed into the community. Pastors often spent time visiting their congregations in their homes, and even though we weren't members of Hawkins Church, Grandma invited Reverend Rossman to meet me and my parents. She came by our home for the first time shortly before Christmas.

I was unsure what to expect. Most ministers I'd known were men who seemed too busy to spend much time with younger people, and I always felt inferior in their presence. Sometimes these men seemed far removed from my generation, coming across as rigid and judgmental, which didn't make me look forward to Sunday services.

Etta entered my world and changed how I felt about ministers. She shared tales about growing up as one of twelve siblings in a Virginia Appalachian Mountain town called Pulaski, located in the western part of the state. She had a medium build and short dark hair, but her unassuming appearance belied her extraordinary personality. She was a captivating speaker and one of the few preachers I'd ever meet whose sermons never felt long enough.

Etta would tell me years later, "Bryant, I admit that I was hesitant to meet you because I wasn't sure how to behave around someone with a disability. But you put me at ease so that soon I didn't even notice the wheelchair." This was something I soon learned to expect when meeting people: they often were unsure how to behave around someone with a physical disability. I was always friendly, answering any questions and trying to set them at ease so they could see that people in wheelchairs were ordinary people who didn't need special treatment.

"I realize that if I had continued along the path I was on before the accident, I would not have had a life."

I got to know Etta very well during her visits to our home and soon I considered her a dear friend. She was caring, funny, and curious. I found that like Sally, she was an older woman I could confide in and trust. We discussed everything under the sun, from serious spiritual and emotional matters, like what was important in life and what gave life meaning, to lighthearted banter and jokes.

One day we were discussing why certain things happen and how they affect a person's purpose.

"Do you ever wonder why you were in this accident and paralyzed?" she asked me.

"Well, I did a lot of talking with God right after the accident wondering why this happened to me, and I figured that there must be some kind of purpose for my life because I lived through it. And now that I've had more time to think about it, I realize that if I had continued along the path I was on before the accident, I would not have had a life."

Her eyes glowed with curiosity. "In what way?"

"My life was off track. I had no direction, no purpose. I was going nowhere. And if this hadn't happened to me, I may have never found the track. I may never even have realized I needed to find the track. I might never have realized my purpose. So if it took the accident to get me to this point... well, I wish there had been another way, but at least I got here."

She smiled. "That's beautifully put and very inspiring."

I shared the story of the lightning strike and how it restored my faith. "Until that moment, I was uncertain that God even had a plan for me. But that single strike destroying that single tree was the answer I needed. I knew then that my life had purpose, and I had to trust in God to find it."

"God truly answered your prayer that night," she said. "Not everyone may see it this way, of course, but I believe as you do that this was a message from Him, a sign that your life has purpose."

"I don't know what that is yet, but I'm sure excited to find out," I told her. "My dream is to have a family someday, so I hope that's in God's plan for me too."

"So do I," she told me with a smile.

On another visit, I told her, "I'm not going to let my disability get me down. I think in life you have to decide whether you're going to work with what you've got or give up, and I definitely don't want to give up. My family and friends are rooting for me and helping me so much, and I'm not going to let them down by giving up on myself after all they've done for me."

"That's exactly the right attitude to have," she

encouraged me. It turned out that Reverend Rossman was dealing with cancer for the second time in her life, so she too was determined not to let her situation defeat her. My positive attitude, despite the challenges my disability presented, inspired her in beating the cancer the second time. Even though in later years it returned more than once, she continued to fight it and get well. I was glad that sharing these conversations helped both of us on our respective life journeys.

The urine that had built up in the tube suddenly splashed loudly into the jug. "What the hell was that?" she exclaimed.

We didn't always have deep, philosophical conversations. We each had a good sense of humor, so we also loved to chat about light-hearted topics and match wits. During one of her first visits, she was sitting in my room and I was lying in bed when I suddenly felt that I was going to urinate. I always wore a Texas catheter, a device that was like a condom with a tube that was affixed to my body with a special body adhesive. The tube emptied into a bag, but when I was home, my parents often substituted an empty milk jug for the bag.

I hadn't ever explained these logistics to Etta so when the urine that had built up in the tube suddenly splashed loudly into the jug, she jumped up with a yelp. "What the hell was that?" she exclaimed.

I couldn't answer her; I was laughing uncontrollably. When I was finally able to catch my breath, I explained what happened.

She dropped back into her chair in relief. "I had no idea what was going on." She gave me a look. "Don't tell anybody I cussed!"

"Uh huh, right," I teased. Her very human response to my situation was a refreshing thing to see in a minister. There was nothing stodgy or unapproachable about her. I saw her as a friend first and a minister second.

My bond with Reverend Rossman always remained strong. After thirteen years at Hawkins Church, she left to become the chaplain at a women's prison, where she worked for seventeen years. Everyone in the community was sad to see her go, but we stayed in touch with letters and Christmas cards and the occasional phone call.

When we said goodbye before she left for her new position, I told her, "Etta, you're the most inspiring preacher I've ever met, and I want you to promise to do two things for me. I want you to marry me if that time ever comes and bury me when that time comes."

"I promise," she agreed with a smile.

Before I knew it, it was graduation day. I'd completed all my coursework with straight A's and would be attending John Tyler Community College in Chester, Virginia. My friends Jamie and Walter would be attending as well. Jimmy had decided to get a job instead of attending college. I'd miss having him around every day but knew that college wasn't for everyone—until the accident, I hadn't been destined for it either.

My parents were very proud of me for graduating

with good grades and going to college, especially my mother. Mom and Dad unconditionally supported me no matter what decisions I made, but Mom always wished I'd go to college like she had. Now I'd be fulfilling her dream, getting a computer degree that would hopefully launch my career.

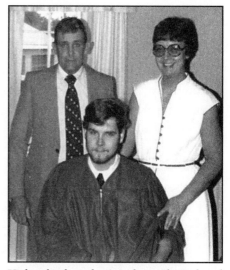

High school graduation day with Dad and Mom—straight A's and going to college!

Graduation day was a bit awkward because I couldn't walk with my classmates into the ceremony. It was held on the football field, and the seniors filed down the steps through the bleachers and out to their seats on the field. I had to wait in the front row for everyone to join me. I was nervous sitting alone in this huge space, but my excitement over my future and the knowledge that my whole family was there to cheer me on helped calm my nerves.

After we received our diplomas and the ceremony ended, the whole family went back to my Aunt Betty's house for a party. I was excited to spend the summer with my friends. Last summer I'd been working hard in rehab, and now I finally had three months all to myself. My friends and I planned a weekend trip to Fishersville to visit my "family" at Woodrow Wilson and rented a motel room near the center. I'd kept in touch with the staff through letters and occasional phone calls, and I couldn't wait to see them again.

It would be the first time I was away from my parents overnight since I'd returned home, so I was excited to test out this bit of freedom. My mother taught my friends how to handle my personal needs and double-checked that we had loaded everything into the van before we departed.

It was fun being at Woodrow Wilson as a guest rather than a patient. Everyone was eager to hear how I'd fared after leaving rehab, and they were all impressed and proud to hear that I'd graduated with honors and would be attending college. They asked after my parents, Grandma Neville, and Steen and Pa.

This was my first time seeing Sally since leaving Woodrow Wilson nearly a year earlier. By now it was clear to me that Sally and I didn't have a future together as I'd once imagined. We lived several hours apart and being with my peers made the age difference seem even wider. Besides, I'd decided that romance needed to be on the back burner while I focused on getting my degree and finding a job.

Sally had shown me such caring and compassion during a time of intense emotional pain, leading my teenage brain to see our friendship as something more. She saved me from spiraling into a deep depression, and I'd be forever grateful, but did that mean she was destined to be my partner? Having spent months outside the insular world of Woodrow Wilson, I now could see that our lives were on different paths. Would she feel the same way?

I asked if we could speak privately. "Of course, Bryant," she said, smiling. "What's on your mind?"

"I've been thinking about what I said to you before I left here last fall—when I told you I was going to make something of myself and come back for you."

"I remember that."

"Well... I still care about you a lot, but now that I've been away from here and back home with everyone, I just wonder... I mean, uh... things are just..." She reached over and took my hand.

"Bryant, when you left here you believed in your feelings at that time. I wouldn't have dared discourage that, and believe me when I tell you how nice it made me feel and how much a part of me wishes it could be. But your life is just beginning and you'll find that special gal one day—you are way too special a person not to have all your dreams come true. You don't owe me any explanations."

She understood! In fact, she had known all along what it took me months to see. I felt a little embarrassed about my misplaced teenage affections, but I was relieved.

"Sally, you'll always be a special friend to me. Can we always stay in touch?"

She grinned. "Of course! If we didn't stay friends, I'd be pretty mad at you. I'm very proud of you, Bryant. You're going to go far in life."

On Sunday afternoon, we said our goodbyes, with promises to keep writing and good-luck wishes for when I started college in the fall. How impressed everyone was with my progress encouraged me.

The only bad part about our trip was that I caught

a cold. It was particularly miserable because it took me a month to get rid of it. It was hard for me to cough and get rid of the congestion, so that darned cold just lingered. Thankfully, I avoided it turning into pneumonia and requiring hospitalization—I didn't want a repeat of my experience in the ICU.

Being home in bed recovering gave me time to think. I was relieved that Sally and I could remain friends without a romantic future, and I was determined to make her proud.

I'd also entirely gotten over my lingering feelings of animosity toward Amy. Even though she'd broken my heart and then further hurt me by dating Steve, I wanted to avoid holding a grudge. She didn't intentionally set out to hurt me. It was a lot to ask of an 18-year-old girl on the brink of adult independence to be with a paralyzed boyfriend for the long haul. We each needed to be free to live our own lives. My decision to shelve my romantic life helped in letting these final negative feelings go. I wasn't focusing on girls, so there was no need to let those from my past weigh on my heart. Amy was my first true love, and I knew she'd always hold a special place in my life. I was sure one day we could even be friends—and eventually as adults, we were.

Once I recovered from my cold, I was able to spend time with my friends again. It was a final, carefree time before we moved into adulthood. I was ready for the challenges and opportunities of college. I didn't know where it would lead me, but I hoped that I would go far.

8
college days

In the fall of 1982 I started at John Tyler Community College in Chester, about an hour from my parents' house. Jamie and Walter were attending too, and we worked out our class schedules so that we'd all be on campus on the same days around the same time. This way they could drive me there and back and help me around the school.

Today John Tyler has expanded to include satellite campuses and larger facilities, but when I attended, it was a small campus of three classroom buildings, with a few classes taught at annexes in Midlothian and at Fort Lee. My classes were all on the main campus so I could get around easily. Walter, Jamie, and I didn't have any classes together though, as I'd decided to study computers, Jamie went for criminal justice, and Walter was undecided. Both knew my schedule and one of them would wheel me from one class to the next. The school was more accessible than my high school—thank goodness, because here I didn't have a team of brawny

— ⚡ —

teenage friends to help me up and down stairs!

The first person I met on campus was my advisor, Mrs. Danztler. Her kindness made me feel instantly welcome and eased my first-day jitters. Over my years at the college, she helped me pick classes and advised me on career options. She inspired me because she had debilitating arthritis and was often in pain but she never complained or let it slow her down.

Despite my computer information systems major, there were some required classes to take first semester, like English and math, before I could get into the computer courses in second semester. I found the atmosphere more serious and focused than high school. Gone were the pranksters and the students who didn't care about their coursework.

Once the professors and students got to know each other, things loosened up a bit and we had some fun, but overall we stayed focused on learning. I enjoyed this as it motivated me to study hard. My strong memory once again served me well as I soaked up every lecture and discussion. My classmates were friendly and none of them seemed to notice my wheelchair or my disability much—they just saw me as another student. This was a relief—I hadn't wanted to stand out or be given preferential treatment.

My teachers made my classes enjoyable and engaging. Dr. Armstrong, who taught statistics, would pass out our exams, then remove his hat and hold it out to us. "Anybody who wants to offer a bribe is welcome to," he'd joke. Mrs. Duty taught English comp and psychology. Her English classes helped me strengthen my writing skills and learn proper grammar, and her psychology classes completely captivated me. I loved learning what made people tick and ended up taking two more psychology classes as electives. I worked hard and got excellent grades in all my college classes, and after my first year I was inducted into the academic honor society Phi Beta Kappa.

I worked hard, got excellent grades, and was inducted into the academic honor society Phi Beta Kappa.

I faced the same challenge I'd had in high school regarding tests and assignments, but the professors helped me find an efficient system for completing my work. A senior student acted as my proctor and filled in my test answers or sometimes Mom came to campus with me to help. But after everyone got to know me and realized I was ethical and wouldn't cheat, I was permitted to take my exams home to complete with Mom's help.

Initially I'd leave my books with the professor, but soon they told me this wasn't necessary. The fact that Mom had been a schoolteacher must have inspired my professors' confidence in my honesty—even if I'd wanted to cheat, I couldn't have gotten anything past a fellow teacher!

Walter left college after only a couple of semesters. It just wasn't for him. He worked in a few different jobs, including general contracting and running an automotive paint business, before finally working for a water treatment systems company in northern Virginia. After he left college, Walter moved into a trailer on my parents' property that had originally belonged to my Aunt Nancy and Uncle George when they were newlyweds. He lived there for several years, and it was a blast having him as a neighbor. He added a ramp so I could get into the trailer and hang out, which I did regularly. I loved having this little degree of independence from my parents' house. Since I was unable to have the college dormitory experience, this was the next best thing.

Jamie continued at college, but he needed to take a job at the sawmill where my father worked to help cover his expenses. We were no longer on similar schedules, so I had to find someone else to drive me to and from school and help me during the day. One of Dad's employees recommended his brother, Bill Roberts, a retired bus driver in his sixties, for the job. Bill was recovering from a heart attack and looking for something low-stress to do.

Bill wasn't just my driver; he became a dear friend. Soon we started fishing together, which I accomplished using a special wheelchair attachment that helped me hold and cast my fishing rod. We also loved sitting together someplace busy and people watching. This was particularly fun at Christmastime, when people got frantic and started acting a little crazy.

Bill had a great time accompanying me to the college. He wasn't idle in the downtime between classes. He was outgoing and loved hanging out in the cafeteria, chatting with students and school employees. Pretty soon he seemed to know more people on campus than I did!

As I completed my computer degree coursework, I took a class in accounting and found that I was a natural. Numbers had always made sense to me, and I liked the rules and precision that came with accounting. My favorite accounting professor was an older woman named Mrs. Haverty. Most people dreaded her classes because she gave hard assignments and was a tough grader, but she was fair and tried to keep class interesting. I found myself with several hours of homework daily in her class, which I actually enjoyed. I liked accounting even more than computers, so I decided to pursue it as a second degree. I completed my computer information systems degree in 1986, and the following year I completed the accounting degree, graduating summa cum laude.

Because few people had home computers at the time, I completed my homework, often in the company of my classmates, in the campus computer labs, using my trusty strap with the pencil. I was good at programming and code and enjoyed helping my classmates with the assignments whenever they got stuck. One student who sometimes needed my help with code work was a woman a few years older than I named Juanita, who I got to know pretty well.

One evening, I was in the hallway outside the computer lab, and a big, long-haired, bearded and tattooed man appeared and headed toward me. I hadn't seen him before, and he looked tough, so I was instantly nervous—what did this guy want with me? The next thing I knew, he sat down next to me. "Hey man. How're you doing? You working in there?" he asked pleasantly, nodding toward the lab.

Who is this, and what is going on here, I wondered.

"Yeah, I am. I'm sorry," I interrupted him. "I don't

think I know you."

"I'm Thom Legacy," he said. "My wife is Juanita. You've been helping her with her computer homework."

A wave of relief washed over me. So this wasn't a Hell's Angel with a bias against guys in wheelchairs!

"Oh, cool! Hey! I'm Bryant," I said, smiling.

"I know. Juanita has told me about you, so I feel like I know you already. Thanks for helping her."

As we chatted some more, I learned that Thom too was working on his degree at John Tyler while working as a field service technician for a company that was eventually bought by Honeywell. He maintained the process and quality control systems in industrial plants that made paper, tires, plastics, and aluminum. We also learned that we shared a love of watching NASCAR races. After that night I started seeing him more around the campus, and we became good friends.

He and Juanita invited me to his graduation party. Their house was in a cul-de-sac and to reach his back yard, I had to go up a steep, bumpy driveway and across some unpaved ground. We had a heck of a time getting my wheelchair up there, but I was glad we made it because I had a great time meeting his family, who were visiting from New England. His brothers were a riot. As we sat around chatting and having beers, his brother Jeff suddenly reached over and swatted their other brother, E.J., across the forehead so hard that E.J. fell out of his lawn chair. Dazed, E.J. looked up at Jeff in confusion.

"Mosquito," Jeff said with a grin.

I laughed so hard I thought my sides would split. I loved the brothers' playful camaraderie and hoped to hang out with them again, even though Thom's driveway had nearly been the death of me.

The next time Thom invited me to visit, I braced myself for another treacherous ascent up his driveway. Instead I found that he and his neighbor had cleaned up the driveway and extended it all the way to his backyard, where he had poured a pad of concrete so my van could back up all the way to the deck.

I couldn't believe Thom had done this for me. Certainly these improvements helped everyone visiting his house, but he'd really done it to make my visits easier. He clearly wanted to be my friend for the long haul and I was touched.

As I spent more time with Thom and Juanita, I got to know their kids, Tanya, who was 11, and Geoff, who was 9. They loved spending time with us, especially Tanya, who always wanted to stay up late playing cards. She was eager to help me with any little thing, like holding my cards or opening doors. I suspected that she might have a crush on me, which was confirmed when she told me she would marry me someday. I always chuckled when she told me this—I was flattered that she liked spending time with me.

Shortly before I got my computer information systems degree, the president of the college, Dr. Freddie Nicholas, approached me on campus to introduce himself. "Hello, Bryant. I'm Dr. Nicholas. I've heard about you from some of the staff and wonder if you'd like to join me for lunch."

"Nice to meet you," I said. "I'd be glad to join you."

Dr. Nicholas was a friendly and approachable man who took a real interest in getting to know the students. I was honored that despite his busy schedule he took

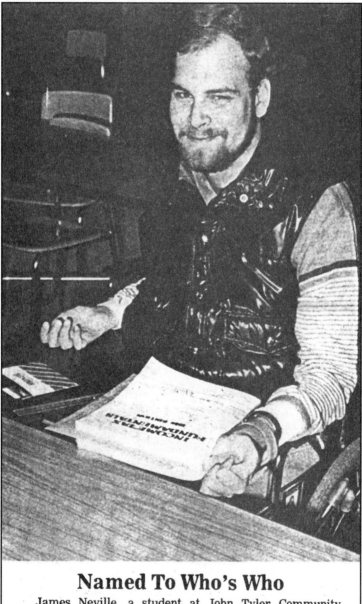

Named To Who's Who

James Neville, a student at John Tyler Community College, has been named to Who's Who Among Students in American Junior Colleges.

time to have a one-on-one conversation with me, and he always stopped to chat for a few minutes whenever he saw me on campus.

After graduating with my second degree in 1987, I spent a few months working as a representative for Dinwiddie County on the foundation board of the college. That summer, Dr. Nicholas recommended me for a computer lab teaching assistant position at John Tyler. I'd only attended one meeting of the board when I got the call that they wanted to hire me. I was happy to get back to the college—I liked the faculty and staff and was able to put my computer skills to use helping students.

Years later, I learned that Dr. Nicholas had been instrumental in helping me get my job when he told me, "I told them that they should hire you because you were such a good student you'd have to be a heck of an employee." Surely it would have been easier for the college to hire someone without a disability—there weren't yet any laws prohibiting discrimination against the disabled in the workplace—but Dr. Nicholas convinced them to see my abilities rather than focusing on my disability.

I always greeted Dr. Nicholas on campus, but even though I was now his colleague I didn't spend much time with him. I soon learned the rigid pecking order of academia meant a lower-level employee couldn't be seen taking up much of the president's time. Adjusting to this bureaucracy was difficult, but it was outweighed by my work helping the students in the labs.

I couldn't teach full time since I didn't have a graduate-level degree, but I got to teach a few special short-term computer courses, including one at my former

Handicapped grad will get diploma standing tall

By LARRY MINKOFF
P-I Staff Writer

CHESTER — James Bryant Neville Jr. may be confined to a wheelchair when he receives his diploma during John Tyler Community College's commencement next Friday. But he will still stand just as tall as the rest of the graduating class.

Neville will receive an applied science degree in computer programming. The 21-year-old quadriplegic will be graduating Summa cum laude, having completed his major with a 4.0 grade-point average.

It took the DeWitt native three years at Tyler to come this far, and, according to Neville, it took a disabling accident to put him on the path of a college education.

On March 21, 1981, while driving back home late at night, a deer ran in front of Neville's pickup truck, causing him to loose control and strike his head on the inside frame of the truck. He broke two vertebrae in his neck and partially severed his spinal cord.

"The accident did more good than bad," stressed Neville, who sports a neatly-cropped blonde beard and baseball cap.

He explained how before the crash, he was a junior at Dinwiddie High School who made passing grades and "was just drifting along."

"Before the accident, I didn't think making grades were important," he said. "After the accident, I saw how important they are."

But that would be just one of the many changes in his attitude towards life, he pointed out.

"I thought before I got hurt that

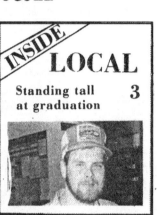

LOCAL

Standing tall at graduation 3

He assured the interviewer that the road to recovery was "hard work," which required between eight to nine hours of painful therapy every day.

Neville returned to finish school, but had missed the chance to apply for college during his senior year. He eventually chose Tyler and said he is glad he did so.

"I have had a lot of teachers here who are top-notch instructors," he noted. "They care about the students, that's not what I expected in college."

Finding college to be much more difficult than he anticipated, Neville said he has spent about eight hours a day attending classes and studying. "It's just like being in a job," he added with a smile.

Explaining that he used to feel awkward when he was pushed into a new class, he said it no longer bothers him.

"I'm of the opinion that if people don't want to understand my condition and would rather stare,

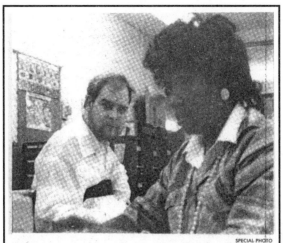

Neville monitors the work of teacher Bettie Perry.

Student has revenge on former teachers

DINWIDDIE — "This is a student's dream," said Bryant Neville, as he started to teach a computer software course in the evenings at Dinwiddie Senior High School. Neville, a former Dinwiddie student, taught the course for Dinwiddie teachers and Central Office Personnel.

There are those who would find teaching one's former teachers intimidating but Neville, who has been a quadriplegic since a high school traffic accident, viewed it as a time to get help and advice from friends.

Although the teachers-turned students were a rowdy bunch and were guilty of enough mischief to exasperate even the most seasoned professional, Neville took it all in good humor. When asked if he would return to do a follow-up course, Neville laughed, "Of course!"

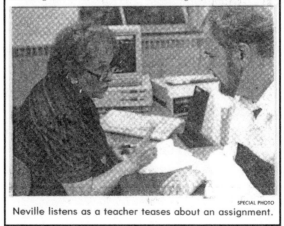

Neville listens as a teacher teases about an assignment.

high school. They had expanded their computer program and the teachers needed help getting accustomed to these new machines, so I gave them some basic lessons. It was a hoot seeing the tables turned: I was the instructor and my former teachers were my students. It reminded me of my daily trip to the teachers' lounge with Jimmy. My teachers were quite proud to see that their former student had two degrees and a full-time job.

Bill Roberts was still my driver, driving me to and from work each day and helping me around campus. Throughout the day, he would park my wheelchair and undo the strap around my chest that helped me sit upright so I could shift my weight around in the seat. The ROHO cushion helped keep my weight shifting so I wouldn't develop pressure sores, but I also had to lean forward and to the sides in my chair.

Soon my colleagues got used to my weight shifting and thought nothing of it, but one day my exercises were particularly memorable. I was suffering from a cold and took a lot of air into my body with all that coughing and sneezing. As one of the ladies from my department stepped into the hall, I leaned forward and let loose the most ungodly loud fart. It was the blast heard down the hall. I didn't even see who was there because she turned and quick-stepped in the other direction.

I heard gasping next to me and saw Bill bent over laughing, slapping the wall in mirth, his stomach shaking. His laughter was infectious, and soon my own laughter dissolved my embarrassment.

"Oh boy, Bryant," he chuckled, righting himself after several minutes. "That lady is NOT going to talk to you anymore!"

Bill teased me about that incident for weeks, and I laughed right along with him. My disability made many of my bodily functions hard or impossible to control, so I learned not to let it upset or embarrass me. I had no place for modesty in my life anymore and knew the best way to set myself and others at ease was to laugh at these incidents. I just felt sorry for the lady who heard my epic blast!

I also couldn't control my bowel movements. Religiously sticking to my bowel program schedule helped reduce the chance of accidents, but they still did happen—always at inopportune times. I could usually tell if an accident was on the horizon. My hair stood on end and beads of sweat formed on my hairline, which meant I'd need to move my bowels within the hour. As soon as I experienced these warning signs, I told whoever I was with, "I have to go!" No questions were asked and it was a race to get me home.

One afternoon Bill was driving me and my great-uncle, Pa, to Richmond to run an errand when I felt those telltale signs. "Bill, I have to go!" He immediately got off the next ramp on I-95 so he could turn around and head back to DeWitt.

"What's going on?" Pa asked.

"Well, Pa, I've got to get home because nature's calling. I don't want to make a mess."

"Got it," Pa said.

As Bill drove the van home, Pa kept turning around and looking at me. "Don't worry, Dick," he said, calling me by my nickname—he had a nickname for everyone. "I believe you're going to make it home."

I did too, but when we were halfway home, my

bowels loosened and the floodgates opened. I watched in horror as my light blue jeans darkened and the van started to smell.

Pa turned around and exclaimed, "Damn, Dick, I believe you've shit!"

"There is no 'believe' about it, Pa!" I said. "I've done it, and it is bad." This was not the first time I'd accidentally soiled myself, but it had never been this bad. It went up my back to my collar and down my pants legs into my shoes. Bill and Pa rolled down the windows and periodically erupted in laughter as the van sped home.

My mother took one look at me and said, "What a mess! How are we going to clean this up?"

"I'll throw him in the pond for you," Dad offered.

I could have been embarrassed at the smelly mess I'd made of myself in front of others, but Bill and Pa treated the escapade as humorous, not horrible. I laughed about it too—there was no point in being upset because it wouldn't help. I just felt bad that my poor parents had to clean me up! I've thankfully never had another accident so bad, but it has gone down as the stuff of legend in our family.

One of the best parts of my full-time job was having a regular salary. I was proud of the income I brought home because I could contribute toward household expenses. My parents had taken such amazing care of me over the years that it felt good to give back and help them in return.

I also enjoyed giving my loved ones surprise gifts and decided to treat Grandma Patsy to a special present.

I arranged a scavenger hunt for her at our house, where she had to read clues and guess where to go next. Once she got to the last clue, I presented her with a tiny box holding a small diamond ring to go with her wedding band. Big Daddy had never been able to afford an

My life was not what I'd imagined before that March night, but now it seemed like exactly where I was meant to be.

engagement ring for her, even though I knew he always wanted her to have one. It was not an extravagant piece of jewelry, and her overjoyed reaction was priceless in comparison.

Big Daddy's spirit had been instrumental in helping me survive my accident and reclaim my life. Giving her such a meaningful gift was my way of thanking them both for being such an important part of my life, both before and after the accident.

Six years after I was injured, I had learned to live with my quadriplegia, had graduated college with two degrees, and was working full-time helping others. Even though I had physical limitations, there was no limit to what I could do with my mind. My life in 1987 was not at all what I'd imagined it would be like back before that March night, but now it seemed like exactly where I was meant to be.

9
banking on the future

I enjoyed working with the students at John Tyler College, but after a year, I realized I wasn't meant to be there long term. I couldn't teach full time without an advanced degree, and the college bureaucracy bugged me. When I found myself begging to run off teaching materials on the copier, I began job hunting.

I submitted resumes anywhere with an even remotely interesting open position. I applied for a computer programming position at the Philharmonic as well as one with the Virginia lottery, which was just launching. I got through two interviews there but they never called with an offer. None of these jobs required physical labor, so I was certainly qualified, but my disability seemed to hinder me. The Americans with Disabilities Act didn't become law until 1990, so it was still legal for businesses to discriminate against disabled applicants and employees. At most interviews, I could tell immediately that there was a bias against me, simply because I couldn't walk.

It was frustrating but I wanted a new challenge and refused to give up. If I kept searching someone was bound to hire me. On days when I felt particularly defeated, I remembered the lightning strike. It was the proof I needed to press on with my search for purposeful work. I was determined to find the right job, so I let friends and neighbors know I was searching.

My second year at the college was complicated by a fire one winter night in one of the classroom buildings. While repairs were underway, the spring semester became a complex dance of moving classes around, holding classes at odd hours, and bringing in trailers as mobile classrooms. Now my schedule was unpredictable, which was inconvenient enough for an able-bodied person but was even more difficult for me because of my personal hygiene regimen. I didn't know how long it would take for things to get back to normal, so I was even more eager to find a job with stable hours.

In June of 1989, Richard Liles, the new president of the local Bank of McKenney, called me with an interesting proposal. He was a member of Bott Memorial Presbyterian Church, so I'd known him my whole life, and he knew I was job hunting. I had helped him with a special computer project at the bank, so he knew my skills.

Steen and Pa were at the house playing cards the night Richard, who went by Dickie, called. "Bryant, the bank needs help creating and managing computer systems. Are you interested in being our computer programmer?"

"I definitely am," I replied, trying to contain my

excitement.

"Now, I can't guarantee how long you'll have a job, and I want you to know that coming in. But I can at least offer you a job right now. Are you still interested?"

"I'm definitely interested, Mr. Liles, even if it's only for a short time. But what do you mean about not knowing how long I'll have a job?"

"I'll explain when you get here. Your cousin Lynda will be working here too, overseeing and modernizing our operations." This was even better news—I'd know someone else on the staff.

Dickie and I discussed a few more details then hung up. I beamed at my family. "I just accepted a job offer with the Bank of McKenney!" Everyone was thrilled. My parents liked the bank because they had accounts there, including their mortgage, and they were happy Lynda would be with me. I was excited because the job would give me more responsibility.

I gave my notice at the college and said goodbye to my colleagues. I would miss them and the students but not the academic pecking order and nit-picky rules. On July 10, I began at the bank with the title of data processing officer. Lynda started the following week—she came from the local Bank of Southside Virginia. After I filled out some paperwork and signed some confidentiality agreements, Mr. Liles handed me a book.

"Now Bryant, the bank is having some problems. You know the former president was fired for embezzlement. As a result, we underwent a Federal Reserve examination. This book contains their findings. It outlines everything, including the non-public details about the embezzlement. It also details all the problems we need to fix. You cannot discuss this outside the bank."

"Is this why you couldn't guarantee me a job for the long haul?" I asked.

"Yes. Depending on how well we can resolve these problems, we may or may not stay open. I have my concerns and want to be up front with you. But I'm determined to work hard and try to keep this place running."

"Me too," I told him.

The embezzlement scandal was a matter of public record and common knowledge in our community. The former bank president had been a nice man, helping many people including my parents, who had gotten an interest-free loan from the bank to pay for my medical expenses. I now learned this wasn't lawful and was a prime example of the bank's lack of compliance with regulations.

The half-inch thick report revealed how the former president had hidden his personal use of the bank's funds through intentionally sloppy record keeping. Before the embezzlement, the bank had about $20 million in assets. Afterward, they had to write off at least a couple of million dollars, which was significant for such a small bank. The former president was jailed and Mr. Liles was hired to try to set the bank straight.

Dickie had previously worked for Bank of Southside Virginia, like Lynda. The Bank of McKenney had been around since 1906 and was the only county bank to survive without a merger during the Great Depression; however, it had never expanded beyond a single branch. I suspected that Bank of Southside Virginia, which had formed through one of these Depression-era mergers, hoped Dickie would resolve the bank's problems so they could buy it as one of their branches. But Dickie didn't just want to sort out the bank's problems to make it attractive to a competitor; he wanted it to thrive independently.

My first year and a half with the Bank of McKenney, we were under a written agreement with the Federal Reserve, which is about as bad as a bank can have it and still be operational. The agreement gave us strict deadlines for implementing policies and procedures. We were a small staff of ten employees with a lot of hard work to do, so we were at the bank seven days a week. That first year we only took Thanksgiving and Christmas days off, but I enjoyed my work. The spirit of camaraderie with my colleagues was a huge motivator.

Although I was working with computers, it was clear that the bank desperately needed an accountant. Each quarter, the bank completed a Report of Conditions and Income, or call report for short. It was like a balance sheet and an income statement that included subsidiary schedules showing the health of the bank overall: its loans, breakdowns of deposit types, and so forth. Mr. Liles wanted us to learn how to do the call report in house. Our second quarter ended June 30 and the call report was filed in July, so one of my first tasks was working with an accountant named Otis, who had been filing the quarterly report for years.

Otis made it clear that the bank wasn't keeping proper records of anything. "How much does the bank have in this type of investment?" He checked the log book and said, "Well, from what's in the book, you have this amount." He scribbled down a figure. "And here are the going rates," he jotted down another figure. "So let's just estimate what you've got."

"What kind of accounting is this?" I asked. Estimating? This was nothing I'd ever heard of—accounting is a precise science. Estimating would not work for a bank, especially one trying to get itself out of hot water with the Fed.

> "'I don't know' worked this time, but don't use that line again. Know what you're doing next time we're here."

I took the report to Mr. Liles. "I know you have no choice but to sign and file this report, but I doubt much, if any, of it is accurate," I cautioned, and explained my concerns over Otis's methods.

That was the last time Otis came around.

A month later, regulators from the Federal Reserve Board, the State Bureau of Financial Institutions, and the FDIC came to do a follow-up exam based on the call report we filed in July to determine whether we were meeting our deadlines and could stay open. They questioned me, but because I was new and confused by Otis's inscrutable methodologies, most of my answers were, "I don't know."

"Okay," one of the regulators finally said. "We appreciate your honesty. 'I don't know' worked this time, but don't use that line again. Know what you're doing next time we're here."

"Will do," I replied nervously. I had a lot to learn! The regulators helped me get a handle on the bank's assets and liabilities, the starting point for building our accounting system. The other employees helped me too, especially our loan officer, Ruth, who gave me a crash course on the banking industry. After weeks of intense examination by all three regulatory agencies, they agreed to let us remain open. By then we had most things close to or in balance.

In addition to keeping the new computer systems running, I helped draft policies addressing our problems. The bank hadn't previously written down its official policies, so we had to prove we could prevent fraud in the future. By the end of the process we had produced seven three-ring binders, each at least two inches thick, full of documentation on our policies and plans.

Now I was in charge of keeping the books. I ensured that we had set up systems that managed every asset and liability, tracked the amount we had, showed what we needed to pay when, and so on. We built these systems onto either our mainframe or the microcomputers. The only estimating was on things like reserves for loan losses, which is acceptable in the industry. Our new mission was to do everything with precision, which paid off.

After eighteen months, we finally got the all clear from the Federal Reserve. We were so proud. It was then that one of the regulators confessed to us, "We actually flipped a coin to see whether or not we'd let your bank stay open, because you were in such a bad state. But you all looked like you wanted a chance to save it, so we gave it to you."

I was glad they did, because I had found my niche. Coming in every day didn't feel like work to me, even on the days when we stayed late or skipped a weekend or holiday. It gave me a sense of purpose to know that I'd been instrumental in helping save this institution, and I was proud that I'd thrived. Dickie had seen past my wheelchair and realized that I had a strong mind and a good personality and he'd given me a chance. I felt loyal to him and the bank, and I wanted to stay and see what happened next.

After the Federal Reserve cleared us, I officially transitioned from computers to accounting. Lynda had experience with computers in her operations job and took over. There was a lot of overlap between the computers and accounting in my new position but I was happy to be working primarily with numbers. Sometimes I marveled at the fact that I happened to have degrees in the two areas of expertise the bank needed most. I was definitely in the right place at the right time. Hard work was rewarded at the bank, so I soon started to climb the ladder of seniority.

Dickie has always been a wonderful boss. A classic type-A personality, he always seemed to be doing two things at once. He also hated confrontation and did his best to keep his employees cheerful with minimal office rules, but initially some people took advantage of this. One of the things that irked Dickie was people not cleaning up the lunchroom. One Saturday, Dickie found dirty dishes everywhere and a sink full of discarded string beans, so he called a meeting that Monday morning.

"Folks," he said, trying to be pleasant, "we need to discuss how the kitchen is always left a mess. Please clean up after yourselves."

As he spoke, several people ignored him, chatting privately among themselves. Dickie then explained a new process we'd be implementing. One of the tellers protested: "We should vote on it."

This was the final straw.

"That's it! I've had enough. This is not a democracy. A lot of you seem to think that, but I'm here to tell you it is not. This is a business, and right now I'm in charge.

"The first thing I want is for every one of us to keep the kitchen clean. The sink was full of dirty dishes and string beans this weekend and I will not tolerate it any longer! Now, as far as the new process, we *will* be implementing it. No voting. Any questions?"

Mr. Liles's Great String Bean Democracy speech, as I affectionately named it, had everyone's attention that day, and from then on, everyone whole-heartedly respected him. Never again did anyone ask to vote on a new process or leave a dirty dish or errant string bean in the kitchen.

During my time at the bank, Bill Roberts had continued to drive me to and from work in my van, but in 1992, he died of cancer. It was a terrible blow to lose my dear friend. It also left me in a quandary: who would drive me to work?

My friend Jamie had some free time and offered to drive me. After a few weeks, the bank offered him part-time work as a gofer. His criminal justice studies in college and a brief stint with the Chesterfield police paid off, because the bank needed someone to handle security, so after a year he was hired full time. He kept up with the constantly changing and often confusing world of banking regulations, ensuring that we avoided problems by staying on the straight and narrow path. Now he's one of the bank's vice presidents and manages our security. Jamie also has an artistic streak and designed the bank's logo.

Mr. Liles's Great String Bean Democracy speech had everyone's attention that day.

In 1992, the Bank of Southside Virginia struck. They applied for permission to buy up to 20 percent of the bank's stock and started aggressively soliciting our shareholders about buying their stock in the bank. But our shareholders were loyal. Many of them were the children or grandchildren of the bank's original shareholders and they wanted to see the bank stay, so stay we did. Bank of Southside Virginia eventually dropped down to owning only 8 percent of our stock.

During this time, we were ready to expand to better serve the community and applied to open our first branch. A second branch followed a few years later. During that time, my career continued growing. I was promoted to controller, and several years later, I was promoted to chief financial officer and senior vice president. Today the bank has seven branches, and we have long-range plans to open more. We went from nearly closing to becoming one of the most respected banks in the state.

I worked hard but always made time for my family and friends. I joined the local chapter of the Ruritan Club, a national men's community service organization that was founded in Suffolk, Virginia, in 1928. The club is similar to organizations like the Lions' Club or

Masons. Once a month we meet and share a meal while discussing how we can fundraise to meet community needs. We've built a community center and are in the process of creating a baseball field. I've twice served as president and also spent several years on their board. I'm also active with Bott Memorial Church. After Steen passed away in 1994, I took over her duties as church treasurer, a position I still hold.

One of my favorite hobbies is attending NASCAR races, which I try to attend several times a year. My best friend, Thom, also loved racing. His brothers and children also loved NASCAR, so going to races often turned into a big family affair. By now Tanya was a young lady and a real pleasure to know. At races she often sat with me in the special seating section for people with disabilities while Thom and the others sat elsewhere.

Early in 2000, I was chatting with one of the bank board's directors, Rudy Hawkins. "I'd love to go to Speed Week and see the Daytona 500 next February," I told him. I knew Rudy's relative worked with the International Speedway Corporation and I thought he might be able to help me get decent seats.

"I'll see what I can do," Rudy told me.

I saw him again numerous times that year, but he never mentioned the Daytona tickets, and by November I couldn't handle the suspense any longer. Planning a trip to Florida would be quite an undertaking, so I asked, "Any word from your relative?"

Rudy smiled. "I've got you covered, no problem! I'll get you the tickets soon." In January of 2001, he gave me 10 tickets and a handicapped parking pass numbered 001.

"Thanks so much, Rudy! What do I owe you for the tickets?"

He shook his head. "Don't worry until you return. We need to be sure those are decent seats!"

I was crushed by Dale Earnhardt, Sr.'s death. His life story inspired me in my own journey.

We booked some hotel rooms for our weeklong trip. Thom made the twelve-hour drive with me in the van, with my parents and E.J. flying down to join us and Jeff and his wife, Marilou, who were both tractor trailer drivers, arriving in their truck. I'd never been to the Daytona 500, and we found out we had the best seats imaginable.

We were all huge Dale Earnhardt, Sr., fans—he had always been a hero of mine, so I was excited to see him race. I admired his passion for racing and his lifelong determination to follow his dream, no matter what obstacles or discouragements he faced. His life story inspired me my own journey dealing with quadriplegia's challenges.

During the Daytona 500 race, Dale crashed in the final lap and was seriously injured. A few hours later he was pronounced dead. Everyone was shocked, especially E.J. and Jeff. They were so upset that they left the track and walked several miles back to our hotel. I was crushed by the death of one of my heroes but knew he left behind a great legacy—including his son, Dale Earnhardt, Jr., who also races cars. Despite Dale's death, we had a great time on the trip.

When I returned I wanted to settle up with Rudy.

—⚡—

"Will you tell me now what I owe you for those tickets?"

He ignored my question and instead asked his own: "Were the tickets any good? Did you have fun?"

"Absolutely!" I enthused. "The seats were amazing and everyone had a blast. If Dale hadn't been killed, it would have been the perfect week."

Rudy smiled. "Paid in full."

I was flabbergasted. "No way! My friends and I want to pay you back. We never expected otherwise."

"I know, Bryant, but you work hard and do a good job. You've never let your disability stop you. I've been blessed to build a good business, but I got help from others when I was just getting started. This is a way for me to pass along what I learned years ago. I believe what goes around comes around. One day you'll find someone who needs your help, and that way you can pay me back."

I've never forgotten Rudy's gift or the lesson he taught me, and I hope I've been able to pay him back many times over since then.

In 2000, I purchased a vacation house on Kerr Lake in North Carolina and also got a 30-foot pontoon boat that was wheelchair accessible. My neighbors on Kerr Lake are a couple named John and Anne, who live there year-round. Shortly after I bought the house, they invited my family and me to a Fourth of July barbecue at their place. We arrived on the pontoon, but I couldn't get onto his dock and up to his house. I didn't mind—someone brought me a plate and I enjoyed the festivities from the boat, but this clearly bothered John and Anne.

Thom explained the accessibility issues with their dock. Even though the world has become far more accessible for those with disabilities, I accept that there are still some places my chair can't go—but John couldn't. When we came to the house the following week, he called me over.

"Bryant, I want to show you something. Let's go down to the dock."

When we arrived, he showed me how he had smoothed out his dock and added a ramp at the end so I could get on and off my boat. I was touched. I'd just met John and he'd made the changes in a week. It reminded me of Thom's kindness in modifying his driveway. From then on we were good friends, and he and Anne sometimes visit us in Virginia and attend NASCAR races with us.

In 2002, the bank sold stock and subsequently had more shareholders than would allow us to stay private, so we had to become a public company. Since this happened after the Enron and WorldCom scandals, publicly traded companies now faced numerous restrictions and requirements, including the most ominous section of law referred to as SOX, after its sponsoring legislators, Senators Sarbanes and Oxley. What a nightmare! But we were determined to meet all of the obligations, so we brought in independent auditors to document our control structure as mandated by SOX.

We were ready by the end of 2003, but things were delayed until 2004. A lot changes in a year, so we had to spend more money to prepare a second time. We were delayed repeatedly, so in the summer of 2009, the bank's board took advantage of a Virginia law that grouped smaller shareholders into a preferred class, allowing the bank to remain private.

Because of my additional responsibilities during this time, I was promoted to executive vice president and Lynda became the senior vice president. I'm proud of my achievements. Nothing was ever given to me except a chance—after Dickie hired me, I had to work hard and prove I was capable of more responsibility. He was willing to see past my wheelchair and give me a chance, and I've proven that he made the right choice.

After I was promoted to a senior officer at the bank, the company gave me a specially equipped van, so I went to the DMV with my assistant, Michelle, to get a handicapped license plate. I learned that the only company-issued vehicles that could get plates were emergency response vehicles, so I filled out the paperwork for a rearview mirror placard.

The clerk looked it over then said, "Everything here seems to be in order. Now take this form to your physician to certify your disability, then we can issue the placard."

I started at him in disbelief. "Look at me! I'm in a wheelchair, I can't move my legs, and my fingers are atrophied. Isn't it clear that I have a disability? You can't do anything by common sense?"

He explained patiently, "Sir, we can't make that judgment on our own. We have to follow the rules."

"All I can say is that the people who employ you don't give you much credit!"

The DMV continued to plague me. My ID card expired and post-9/11 security was tight. It seemed I'd need an act of God to get my new ID.

A clerk at the DMV reviewed a list of documents

they would accept as proof of my identity. "Are you a vet? Married?" she inquired.

"No to both," I replied.

She continued down the list of documents I didn't have until she finally said, "Here's one we can use: your welfare card."

Her assumption that I was on welfare because of my disability irked me.

"We can't, ma'am, because I don't have one!" I snapped. Her assumption that I was on welfare because of my disability irked me. I knew some people genuinely needed welfare and other social services, but the only public assistance I'd ever received was a small gasoline stipend while I was in college. I'd never been on welfare and hoped I never would be. I was able to use my birth certificate and school transcripts to get my new card, but learned another valuable lesson: never let your ID expire.

Some people I met had completely missed the memo on political correctness. Every year, the area Ruritan Clubs holds an event in Emporia, Virginia, called the Pork Fest, where people get together and cook pork in numerous ways. One year when I arrived in my van with Thom, we pulled into a parking area reserved for dignitaries and people with disabilities. An older gentleman hurried over and threw up his hands.

"Stop! You can't park here, this is reserved."

Thom leaned out the window and explained, "I've got a man in a wheelchair, so we need to park here." He pointed at my mirror placard.

The man peered into the window. "Oh, you got a cripple in there? Come on up here!"

As he directed us into the parking spot, Thom said, "That old dude just called you a cripple, Bryant." We chuckled.

As we prepared to cross the road to the festival, the older man walked into the middle of the street, threw up his arms to stop traffic, and yelled, "Cripple in the road! Cripple in the road! Come on through here, son. We take care of our cripples in Emporia."

We stifled our laughter until we were out of earshot. Instead of getting offended, I was actually touched. Despite his language, this man had gone out of his way to help me. His intentions were good, so I hadn't the heart to correct him—I knew he hadn't called me a cripple out of malice.

The people I do have trouble with are wait staff. Most waiters and waitresses seem uncomfortable around me and often avoid addressing me directly. Usually the waitperson asks someone with me, "What would he like to eat?"

"I don't know," my companion replies, "why don't you ask him?" I always try to be polite and empathetic, figuring that the poor waiter or waitress assumes that I might also have a mental disability. They usually relax after I talk to them, but it's uncanny how often this happens.

After the Americans with Disabilities Act passed in 1990, the world gradually became easier to navigate. Sidewalks had ramps for wheelchairs, parking lots were required to have designated handicapped spaces, and even buildings became easier to get around, with elevators, wider hallways, and automatic doors. Even the terminology changed, evolving from being a handicapped person to being a disabled person to being a person with a disability. This new phrasing makes it clear that the disability is just a part of me as opposed to being what defines me.

My colleagues don't think of me as a person with a disability anymore. Sometimes if we're planning an off-site meeting or event and I bring up accessibility questions, they'll say, "I forgot about your wheelchair!" This is one of the most flattering compliments anyone can pay me, because it means they see me as Bryant, not as a man in a wheelchair. I've never wanted my wheelchair to stand in my way, but I've also never wanted it to accord me preferential treatment.

"I forgot about your wheelchair!" is one of the most flattering compliments anyone can pay me.

In 2003 I switched to an electric wheelchair. I hadn't used one since rehab and knew it would give me more independence, especially after buying the lake house. The manual chair had helped me to keep up the strength in my arms, and having a companion push me around was a treat. But now I used my upper body often at work and there was no need to use the manual chair for exercise.

What a huge difference the electric chair made. I was dependent on others for so many things in my life, so it was wonderful to do something as fundamental as moving from room to room on my own. Electric chairs had improved a great deal since I used one in the early

1980s, so it was pretty easy to get used to my new chair, which had a joystick on the arm for navigation and a lap tray that could be attached to help me eat and drink and carry things. I still occasionally bump into things or people, but it's mostly smooth sailing. Now I can't imagine life without it.

Some people look at a wheelchair as a confinement but I don't. My wheelchair gives me the freedom to move and takes the place of my legs. It allows me to "walk" using wheels instead of my feet. It only enhances my quality of life. When I was first injured, I often awoke from dreams where I'd been walking. Now when I dream I'm always in my wheelchair. It has become a part of me.

> Now when I dream I'm always in my wheelchair. It has become a part of me.

10
filling the void

When I turned 37, things were great. My life was full of trips to the lake house, NASCAR and NHRA/IHRA races with friends, events with the Ruritan Club and in my community, and the bank's expansion, but I still felt a void. The only thing missing was a family of my own. My dearest dream eluded me, by my own doing. I'd shelved my romantic life while I pursued my education and career. Now I'd exceeded my own expectations and my life was a success. It was time to find someone to share it with.

This was easier said than done. I felt too old to try the bar scene and would have been a third wheel going with another couple, like Thom and Juanita. I couldn't think of other options for meeting new people so I decided to try online dating. Nowadays many people have great success finding romance on the web, but when I tried it in 2000 it wasn't very popular. I didn't want to tell my friends I was online dating—my first clue that it wasn't right for me—but I signed up for several sites.

I met a few ladies online who seemed okay, but nothing developed with them.

Finally I met a nice woman named Christine, who went by Chris. She lived in St. Louis, Missouri, and after exchanging emails and chatting on the phone, we agreed to meet. She came to visit me several times at Kerr Lake and we really hit it off. She seemed to care about me and my disability didn't faze her. After a few months I decided to invite her to DeWitt for the weekend to meet my family—and so I could propose.

That Saturday we went to a restaurant with my parents, Thom and Juanita, and their children, Tanya and Geoff, who were now grown. Earlier I had presented Chris with a ring and my proposal, which she excitedly accepted. When we got to dinner, she showed off her ring and we received lots of congratulations and well wishes. Chris and I had only known each other a few months, but I was convinced that she was the right woman for me.

It turns out she wasn't. Several hours after dinner, Chris and I argued—I've tried hard over the years to remember why—and she returned the ring, storming out of the house in a huff. I must hold the record for the world's shortest engagement. I was so annoyed I wanted to return the ring the next day but had to wait until the store opened on Monday. My parents and friends seemed secretly relieved things hadn't worked out—I had been in such a rush to propose that I hadn't taken the time to really get to know Chris.

I feared ending up alone and kept looking for love, but clearly I hadn't learned my lesson, because where did I go? Back online. I tried eHarmony, which finds your ideal mate for you, and it rather depressingly came up with zero results. I had a few more unsuccessful dates using other sites before I decided this was not the avenue for me. If I was fated to find a partner it would

Part of me wanted to find out if Tanya had feelings for me, but the other part was hesitant to push the issue.

happen in real life, no matter how long it took.

During this time, I noticed that Thom's daughter, Tanya, seemed friendlier than usual. In November of 1999, she had given birth to twins, Joseph and Zachary. Tanya had a lot on her plate. The boys' father wasn't interested in being part of their lives, so she was raising them on her own.

Tanya moved into a trailer on my parents' property when the boys were toddlers, so I got to see her and the twins regularly. I enjoyed watching them grow from the day they were born. I didn't have my own nieces or nephews, so it was fun to spoil them. Since Tanya was now our neighbor, I saw a lot of her.

I suspected that Tanya's friendliness was flirtation. She had a crush on me when she was younger and teased me that she would marry me someday, and I had laughed it off. I went so far as to tell her, when she was in her early twenties, that if she was still single at age 30, we could try getting together, but I pointed out that life with me would pose challenges so she should wait until she was older. She had agreed, knowing that the boys would take a lot of her time and energy. I figured she'd

— ⚡ —

settle down with someone her own age, but that hadn't
happened. Now she was nearly 30, so I started wondering
if her playfulness meant she had feelings for me.

Part of me wanted to find out, but the other part of
me was hesitant to push the issue. Tanya had her hands
full with the twins and it didn't seem fair to add in the
possibility of caring for me. Then there was the matter
of her father. Thom was my best friend and I didn't
want to put our friendship in jeopardy by pursuing his
daughter. If Tanya and I did get together and things
didn't work out, I knew I could stay friends with both
Tanya and Thom, but he might worry that it would strain
our friendship. And I knew my own parents worried
about my future partner caring for me. It was not a
responsibility to be taken lightly.

I continued in this state of uncertainty about Tanya
for a couple of years. We were great friends, so it was
hard to transition to thinking about her as a potential
love interest. But around Christmas of 2005, something
happened that made me decide to take the plunge and
learn her intentions.

Thom and his family were at the lake house for a
weekend visit. After the twins had gone to bed and her
mom and dad were watching TV in the next room, Tanya
and I stayed up late playing cribbage in the kitchen. I
kept getting good hands and winning, so I teased her.

"Oh, just bite me," she said with a grin.

I gave her a surprised look. Where had this come
from?

I beat her again, and once again she said, "Bite me,
Bryant!"

"Watch out now," I joked. "If you keep saying that, it

might happen."

When I beat her in yet another game, she said it a third time. "Bite me, Bryant!"

It was midnight and her father came in. "You going to bed tonight, dude?" He needed to help me get into bed

"You know, you don't walk the walk," she said. I grinned. "What are you saying, that I'm crippled?"

and obviously wanted to go to bed himself, so I said goodnight to Tanya. As I lay in bed, I turned her words over in my head. She had seemed flirtatious, but I just couldn't be sure.

The next morning, Tanya and I sat together on the porch, and I was teasing her about something. She turned to me and said, "You know, you talk the talk, but you don't walk the walk."

"What are you saying, that I'm crippled?" I grinned.

She looked at me seriously. "That has nothing to do with it."

My head spun. Was she implying that I was willing to flirt with her but not take any action? After we got home from the lake, I had a heart-to-heart with Thom.

"Thom, I need to ask you about Tanya. You're usually around when we're together. Does it seem to you like she's flirting with me?"

Thom thought for a moment. "Now that I think about it, yes it does."

"I need to find out how she feels for sure," I said. "This has been going on for a while and I just want to know. I'm no good at romantic games."

I wrote her a letter saying just that: I was no good at games. Was she flirting with me? Writing to her was easier because I figured it would be too difficult and potentially embarrassing to talk in person. I put the letter in a Christmas card, along with her gift: tickets to a drag race. Then I sent it and waited.

We were all scheduled to go back to the lake house for New Year's Eve, but Tanya was staying home with the boys, who were grounded for misbehaving. My chance to talk to her came on the Friday night before Christmas, when she and her family joined me for dinner at a Japanese restaurant. I had sent her the card several days prior and was certain it must have arrived. But during dinner she didn't say anything. The only remotely flirtatious interaction we had was when the hibachi chef offered me some extra shrimp Juanita didn't want.

"Hold on now, don't give those all to him!" she protested, laughing and grabbing several shrimp from my plate. But other than that, nothing.

I had a sinking feeling. What if she had read the letter and was surprised that I'd misread her playfulness as something more? What if she didn't have feelings for me? Tanya left the restaurant early to put the boys to bed. I couldn't wait any longer; I had to know her thoughts. Once the rest of us got home from the restaurant, I pulled Thom aside.

"I sent Tanya a card a few days ago with her present inside," I said, trying to sound casual. "Could you go over and check if she received it? She didn't mention it tonight and I'm worried that it didn't arrive."

He agreed and headed over. A few minutes later, Tanya knocked at our door. "I asked Dad to stay with the boys for a few minutes," she said. "I figured I'd come over here and give you a hard time for not asking me about the card yourself." She smiled.

I smiled back, feeling nervous. "Did you get a chance to read my letter?"

"I did."

"What did you think?"

When she pulled back and looked into my eyes, I could tell we had shared a truly magical moment.

"Well, I guess you're right—I have been flirting with you without being direct. But you have been just as guilty."

This was a relief—I hadn't been reading more into the situation. I still didn't know if she actually wanted to take a chance on a relationship. "Well, since you won't be coming down to the lake for New Year's, can I get my kiss early?" I asked.

"Of course," she said. She leaned over and kissed me.

It was magical. Sparks flew—I felt like I was seeing stars. I'd never felt like this kissing anyone before. Until we kissed, I hadn't known if my feelings for Tanya were truly romantic or if it was just deep affection for a longtime friend. But after we kissed, I knew that my love for her wasn't as a friend. I'd fallen in love with her.

When she pulled back and looked into my eyes, I could just tell she felt the same way, that we had just shared a truly magical moment. We spent a little while talking and decided to start officially dating. We agreed it was best not to tell the boys for a while, so we could see where things went.

"No matter what happens with our relationship, we must vow to stay friends," I said.

"I agree."

But I think both of us knew we'd found our soul mate in each other after that first magical kiss.

She told me then how she felt about my short-lived engagement. "When I found out you were engaged to Chris, I thought I'd lost my chance with you, and I was so upset," she admitted.

"Well, I'm sure glad that didn't work out," I said.

"Me too!"

Joseph and Zachary's punishment was lifted, so Tanya and the boys were able to come to the lake house for New Year's after all. I thought 2006 was off to a great start.

But both my mother and Tanya's father were initially apprehensive about our relationship, each for their own reasons. Mom knew what a labor-intensive responsibility my care presented and worried that the boys would keep Tanya too busy to also handle caring for me. After seeing how poorly things had ended with Chris, Mom also didn't want me to deal with more emotional upset if Tanya and I broke up.

Thom was worried about our friendship.

"What happens if you and Tanya split up?" he asked me. "How can we stay friends?"

"Well, Thom, Tanya and I have discussed this, and we want to give the relationship a try. If it doesn't work out, we've agreed that we'll go back to just being friends. I have every intention of doing so, if we part ways, and I have no intentions of ever not being your friend."

"How can you be so sure?" he pressed.

"I'm not one to hold grudges or cause drama, and neither is your daughter. Neither of us wants to hurt you."

Thom seemed skeptical, but as time passed and he realized

"Hey, I raised two boys," Tanya said. "I know about bodily functions. I can manage."

that not only were Tanya and I devoted to each other but also that nothing had changed between him and me as friends, he relaxed and even seemed to enjoy seeing Tanya and me together.

As the months passed, I considered proposing. I had no doubts about marrying Tanya; I loved her and trusted her completely. But I was worried about how she would react when she learned about the specifics of my more intimate personal hygiene routines. She seemed committed to me, so I wanted her to know exactly what she was getting herself into. I had hinted at it but had never discussed the specifics because they'd never been relevant. Now they were.

"Tanya, I want you to know about the personal routines I need help with as a quadriplegic. My mother has done these for me, but if we were to live together or get married, you'd need to handle my catheter and bowel programs."

"I'm ready to learn how to do it," she told me.

"It's not pleasant," I forewarned her.

"Hey, I raised two boys," she said. "I know about bodily functions. I can manage."

I wasn't worried about the catheter, because she'd seen her dad perform the procedure at the lake house, but I was truly nervous about bowel program. It was an involved and intimate process where twice a week, my mother would undress me, lay me on my side, and insert two suppositories, then wait for nature to take its course.

I used to sit on a toilet chair to move my bowels, but years earlier my father had been weakened by a mild stroke, so he could no longer lift me onto the seat. Now Mom placed a disposable pad and pile of paper towels under me to catch and dispose of the waste. The process took three or four hours and was smelly and messy. Afterward Mom cleaned me up and got me dressed again.

It was important for me to stay on my bowel program schedule to prevent any digestive problems. I worried that the unpleasantness would be off-putting to Tanya and wondered if she'd want my mother to keep doing it, or if we'd need to hire an aide.

I didn't give her enough credit. "Bryant, if this is something I need to do to be with you, I'll do it. It doesn't bother me."

I was relieved. "I thought this might scare you off," I admitted.

"Scare me off? I love you, Bryant! Part of loving you is caring for you, and this is part of that, so of course I'll do it."

Over the next year, Tanya learned how to care for all my needs, including the bowel program. She started each new process cautiously, concerned about doing something wrong or hurting me, but she was determined to learn everything. Mom saw her determination too and her concerns diminished. I'd been Mom's baby for 40 years, so seeing her willingly transfer responsibility to

— ⚡ —

another person was a big deal.

I truly felt like the luckiest man alive to have found a partner like Tanya. The fact that she wasn't daunted by my disability's challenges made me sure that she was meant to be my wife. I also loved her sons and already felt like they were my own. I could envision us living together in our own home as a true family.

When I broached the subject of marriage, Tanya seemed enthusiastic but brought up a stipulation.

"There's one thing, Bryant. Joe made me promise I'd wait until I turn 31 to get married."

I chuckled. "Why did he ask that?"

"I'm not sure, but I want to keep that promise," Tanya said.

"All right, I'm happy to wait. We'll get married after you turn 31." This meant waiting until after August of 2007, but that was okay with me. We still had to tell the boys about our relationship, so we decided engagement could wait. I was worried they might be reluctant to share their mother's affection with someone else, even someone they already knew and liked. But in Christmas of 2006, my mind was set at ease by seven-year-old Zachary.

I was with Tanya and the boys shortly before the holiday when Tanya, smiling, prompted Zachary, "Tell Bryant what you asked Santa for this year."

I expected him to list some highly desired toys or games and was heartened to hear him say, "A dad." My heart melted and tears filled my eyes.

"And who do you have in mind, Zach?" I asked with a tremble in my voice.

Without hesitation, he replied, "You."

The waterworks started. I turned to Tanya, sniffling. "Surprise!" she said. She had wanted me to hear Zachary's wish firsthand.

It was clear that the boys accepted me, so we shared with them our news that we planned to officially become a family—once Tanya was 31, of course, which satisfied Joe. I would be able to grant Zachary's wish while granting my own greatest wish of being a father.

I wanted to make a formal proposal and get Tanya a ring—although after my previous proposal experience, I decided to ask first and then make my purchase! I also wanted to make plans to build us a house. My father owned 62 acres of land and since he had general contracting experience, I discussed plans with him for building our own home on his land.

In early June of 2007, I formally asked Tanya to marry me when we were in Rhode Island visiting her relatives for a week, during a moment when we were alone. We were thrilled to be engaged but decided to keep it to ourselves for a few days. Tanya was the kind of woman who didn't want an elaborate proposal and huge ring, but I wanted to make things official with a ring so we could share the news with our family.

My mother's birthday was on June 21, and Tanya and the boys came over to wish her a happy birthday. As the boys headed out, I said, "Wait Tanya, I've got something for you." Earlier that day I'd purchased a diamond ring and had shown it to my mother, who was overjoyed. She didn't know that Tanya and I were, for all intents and purposes, already engaged, and I didn't tell her otherwise because she seemed so excited.

"When are you going to propose?" my mother

demanded.

"So you've gone from not knowing if we should even be in a relationship to wanting to know when we're getting engaged? What a change of heart!"

"I know Tanya is the right woman for you."

Mom had put the ring on my wheelchair tray in the hopes that Tanya hadn't seen it.

Mom was so excited, I decided to give Tanya the ring in front of her.

Mom had put the ring on my wheelchair tray in the hopes that Tanya hadn't seen it, and Tanya, to her credit, played it cool and acted like she had no idea what was going on.

"Tanya, will you look at my tray? There's something there for you." She smiled as she saw the ring. "Will you marry me?"

"Yes, Bryant, I will," she said, slipping it on her finger.

My mother was delighted. It was fun to share the news with the rest of our families too—everyone was happy for us and looked forward to our wedding. No one seemed to doubt that we should be together—and Tanya had been sure about it since she met me as a young adolescent! It made us chuckle that she had correctly predicted that she would marry me someday.

That year, Thom and Juanita sold their home in Chesterfield and moved into a home they built across the road from my parents' house. The neighborhood they'd been living in had gotten quite developed and they wanted a quieter country home experience, so my father gave them five acres to build on. Once my new home was built, I'd be next door to my parents and across the road from my in-laws. Some newlyweds might not want such close proximity to their families, but for us it was a blessing. It was great to have help close by should we need it, and I was pleased that the boys would be near both sets of grandparents.

My father and I made sure to plan the new house with accommodations for my wheelchair. The whole house was built on one floor with a master bedroom, two bedrooms for the boys, and three bathrooms so no one would have to fight over access. We also had a garage large enough to accommodate two cars. The interior and exterior of the house had ramps and sidewalks so I could access every part of it. There was even a small pond on the eastern side of the yard. Construction started in October and the house was completed in April of 2008. It was exciting to watch the progress on the house. I'd finally be moving out of my parents' house after 40 years. I was glad I wasn't going too far, because I loved spending time with my folks, but it would be nice to finally feel physically independent and embark on this new chapter in my life. Finally, after decades of hoping, my dream of having a family would be reality.

The wedding was set for May 24, 2008. We spent several months planning a simple affair in the yard of the Kerr Lake house—neither Tanya nor I wanted a lot of fuss. Thom hired a caterer to serve fried chicken and fixings and my Aunt Mary Katherine offered to make us a wedding cake as a gift. We rented chairs for our guests and invited them to come dressed as casually as they liked. "It's not fancy," we told our friends and family. "Just come dressed comfortably and ready to have fun." The boys would wear suits and I would wear a suit jacket with jeans, which were more comfortable for me than suit pants. Tanya wanted to wear jeans and a T-shirt since she was most comfortable in those, but her brother, Geoff, convinced her to wear a wedding dress. "You'll regret it if you don't," he told her.

"You promised you were going to marry me and bury me." I said. "Now I remember. Which one are you ready to do?"

"I don't think I will," she protested, but she knew it would make her family happy, so she got a simple white gown.

Geoff and his fiancée Rachel would be the groomsman and bridesmaid, my father would be my best man, and Tanya's mother was her maid of honor. The boys would be the ring bearers, each of them carrying one ring up the aisle.

I couldn't wait to call Reverend Etta Rossman. When she answered the phone, I was so excited I didn't even introduce myself.

"Do you remember the promise you made me years ago?" I asked.

"Well, hello, Bryant!" she said. "It's nice to hear from you, but you'll have to refresh my memory on that promise."

"You promised me that you were going to marry me

and bury me."

"Now I remember. Which one are you ready to do?"

I laughed. "I'm getting married this May, Etta, and I'd be thrilled if you would officiate."

"I'd be honored and delighted," she said.

"I'm in no hurry for you to fulfill the other half of your promise, by the way."

The morning of the wedding dawned rainy and overcast. My mother was worried. "The wedding is outside. What will we do if it rains all day?" she fretted.

"Well, I guess we'll just get wet," I replied. I was so excited nothing could upset me. I didn't even feel nervous. By 10 in the morning, the rain had cleared and there wasn't a cloud in the sky. It seemed like the rain had fallen just to settle the dust and refresh the air.

I stayed in Virginia with my parents while Tanya and her family headed down to North Carolina early to get everything ready. After the rain cleared, Tanya and her father set up the folding chairs for our guests. Every now and then, a little gust of wind would shake raindrops from the trees onto them and the chairs. As soon as Tanya and Thom would wipe the chairs dry, the breeze blew more raindrops onto them.

"That's Uncle Jeff," said Tanya. Her uncle had died of cancer almost four years prior, and we all missed him terribly. He had been so full of life and was so much fun to be around, so Tanya was convinced that his spirit was in the yard that day teasing them by shaking the raindrops on their heads. It was just the sort of mischievous prank her uncle would have loved to play.

Uncle Jeff wasn't our only guest who was there in spirit. I was sure all my grandparents were there, along with Steen and Pa. I was certain Pa was helping Jeff mischievously shake raindrops on the chairs. The sun's rays seemed to carry all our loved ones' spirits down to share our joy that day.

Another guest who couldn't attend was Sally. She and I had stayed in touch over the years and I still considered her a dear friend. But by the time I invited her to the wedding in 2008, she was unwell. She suffered from a severe respiratory illness and needed to use an oxygen tank, so she was unable to travel.

She sent me her regards. "I'm sorry I can't be there, Bryant, but I wish you all the best. Please bring your new family to meet me soon." I promised her I would.

My parents and I arrived later in the morning. Everyone went to great lengths to keep Tanya and me from seeing each other before the wedding. I was thrilled to see the chairs in the yard filling with our relatives and some of my closest friends, including Jamie, Walter, and John and Anne. My closest colleagues were there too: Dickie, Michelle, my cousin Lynda, and Ruth.

At one o'clock, we started the ceremony. Etta, my father, and I waited at the end of the aisle under a simple flower-draped canopy. First Geoff escorted Rachel and then Juanita up the aisle, followed by the boys carrying our rings, and finally Tanya walked in on Thom's arm.

When I saw Tanya, my jaw dropped in amazement. Her aunts and future sister-in-law had gotten a hold of her that morning and done a major makeup job as well as styling her long blonde hair, crowned by a white headpiece. Tanya never bothered with makeup and

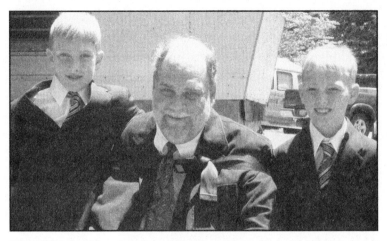
With Zachary and Joseph at the wedding. By marrying Tanya, I fulfilled Zachary's wish for a dad and my wish to be a husband and father.

elaborate hairstyles because she was a self-proclaimed low-maintenance woman, and I didn't think she needed it because to me she was the prettiest woman in the world. Now she looked more beautiful than ever.

Reverend Rossman's ceremony was beautiful, with lots of personal touches—she was able to share some stories from our years of friendship.

There were some laughs during the ceremony too—not all intentional. When she turned to Tanya for her vows, she instructed, "Repeat after me. 'I, Tanya, take this man, James Bryant Neville, Jr., to be my lawfully wedded husband.'"

But instead of pausing, Etta continued reciting the rest of the vows. I looked at Tanya, whose eyes grew bigger with each line. I struggled to contain my laughter—I was next!

Reverend Rossman recovered perfectly. Seeing the terrified look on Tanya's face, she exclaimed, "Oh, Lord,

— ⚡ —

I forgot to pause didn't I?" Our guests laughed. "Do you, Tanya?" she asked.

Relieved, Tanya got off with a simple, "I do."

Then she turned to me, and I figured I'd get the same treatment, but no! I dutifully repeated my vows from start to finish—though this time Etta paused after each line.

After the vows, Etta said to me, "Now you've got two young sons and as their father you are responsible for leading them in their faith journey." I took this vow very seriously and a year later baptized the boys as members of Bott Memorial Presbyterian Church.

We'd decided to include a special task for each of the boys. Since I could not physically put the ring on Tanya's finger, Joseph stood in for me, and Zachary helped Tanya place my ring on my finger. It took a little work, but together they got it over my atrophied knuckle. We had chosen Zachary to put on my ring as a symbol of both our dreams coming true: he got his dad and I got my family.

Reverend Rossman declared us husband and wife, Tanya leaned down and kissed me, and everyone applauded. This was it: we were married! I thought my face would split from smiling so hard. We turned to our guests and were engulfed by dozens of well-wishers.

Once the congratulatory crowd had parted, I said to Tanya, "Honey, you look beautiful, but you know you didn't need to get all done up. You're always beautiful."

Tanya made a funny face. "Well, I didn't want to do it, but my aunts and Rachel made me do it. It made them happy."

Everyone enjoyed the picnic lunch and wedding cake

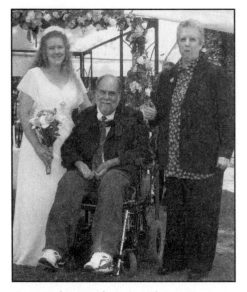

Tanya and me with Reverend Etta Rossman, my dear longtime friend who performed our wedding ceremony.

in the sunshine, then some of our guests stayed with us to open presents. It was a casual, relaxed day and I enjoyed every minute of it. Everyone was genuinely happy for us to be married, even the boys, who were hot and uncomfortable in their suits but so happy that they didn't mind wearing them for a while. Once everyone had taken pictures, they dashed into the house to change.

Our wedding represented my dearest dream becoming a reality: I was a husband and a father. My life felt complete and I knew I had realized my true purpose. I was a family man now.

A couple of months later, I kept my promise to Sally. Her family and friends threw her a surprise birthday party at a community center near her home in Staunton, and I traveled there with Tanya and the boys. It was fun to see old friends from my Woodrow Wilson days, especially R.S., and I enjoyed introducing all of them to my family. But there was a note of sadness to the day too—Sally was frail. Her illness was taking its toll and I knew this would be our last visit together.

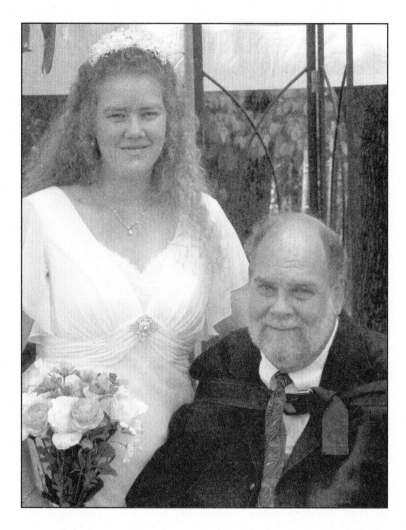

During the party she pulled me aside and quietly told me, "I'm so glad you found the right girl, Bryant. You never knew how much I wished it could have been me long ago, but if it had been, we'd be getting ready to say goodbye to each other."

I knew it was hard for her to speak and even breathe at this point, so her words meant the world to me.

— ⚡ —

"Thank you for everything you did for me, Sally," I told her gently. "You saved me and made it possible for me to be here today, married with sons. I'll never forget how you helped me."

A few weeks later, she was gone.

11
a dream fulfilled

After the wedding we adjusted to our life together as a family in our new home. Early in 2008, Tanya left her job leading a data entry team at a warehouse to be around during the final stages of construction on our home. I always told Tanya that she didn't have to work unless she wanted to, and in the first year of our marriage, it helped that she could focus on learning my care routine. But she was soon bored just staying at home.

Providing for the family on a single income was causing a few cutbacks too, so we were all glad when in March of 2009 she applied for and was offered a job in networking at the Bank of McKenney IT department. Working in the same office made our lives easier, because Tanya could drive me to and from work and help me when needed at the office.

Tanya cared for most of my hygiene needs, but soon Zachary and Joe were pitching in, brushing my teeth, washing my face and hair, and keeping my beard shaved and trimmed. The biggest change came in my relationship with them. I was now their stepfather, so I'd gone from a friendly "uncle" who had enjoyed spoiling them to a parent—which meant disciplining them. The first time I had to holler at them for misbehaving, they shared a look of shock as it sank in that now they'd have to mind me. They were generally good boys, but like all children, they knew how to push their mother's buttons and each other's. Even though parenting could be tough, I did enjoy my new responsibilities and hoped I could live up to Mom and Dad's excellent example.

The only thing that ever saddened me was being unable to participate in the boys' beloved sports activities. They played soccer, baseball, basketball, and football. I wished I could play catch and run around the yard with them, especially since I loved baseball so much as a child, and sometimes when it was very cold outside, I couldn't attend their games. My body was sensitive to temperature extremes, so I had to miss some of their sporting matches to prevent possible health problems. But this was my only regret. Hearing them call me "Dad" or "Daddy" never failed to make me glow a little inside. My parents, too, loved their roles as Grandma Gloria and Grandpa Jimmy and treated the boys as their own grandchildren.

I was grateful to have such a wonderful relationship with my stepsons and planned to legally adopt the boys. They already felt like my own flesh and blood, but I knew the benefits of making them officially my own. The adoption process was arduous and time-consuming, but I was determined to do it.

On our first wedding anniversary, as Tanya and I made plans to go out somewhere special to celebrate,

Zachary piped up.

"Why can't we go?"

"Well, son, this is our wedding anniversary," Tanya explained.

"Yes, but it's our anniversary too. We all became a family that day."

I did still sometimes think about having my own biological child

Tanya and I both melted a little. The things that came out of this boy's mouth! There wasn't much we could say, because he was right. I thought for a moment before responding.

"You're right, it is the day we became a family, and that's special. But this is our first anniversary as husband and wife—it's important so we're going to celebrate this one by ourselves. But we'll take you and your brother out with us on our second anniversary." This satisfied Zachary, and a year later, we honored our promise and took the twins with us. Going out as a family became our annual anniversary tradition.

I did still sometimes think about having my own biological child—from the time I was young this had been my biggest dream. Tanya and I had known each other over twenty years, so she was well aware of my lifelong hopes and dreams. I didn't want to push her into having another baby, but we did broach the subject sometimes before going to sleep. As we neared the holidays in 2009, we had a real heart-to-heart one evening.

"I feel like Zachary and Joe are my own boys, especially since I've always known them, and that is gift enough," I told Tanya. "You don't need to go through having another baby just for me."

"I know, Bryant, but I also know you missed out on so much of the experience of being a dad, the behind-the-scenes things," she said. "You weren't there for everything that comes with raising a baby: the late nights and the diaper changes and watching the baby sit, crawl, and take the first steps. You've always wanted that, and I know it."

"You're right, but you've already given me so much. How can I ask for anything else?"

"I'd like to have a baby with you—I think you should get to have that experience. And I think the boys would like a little brother or sister," she said.

This made me glow inside. She wanted another baby too! "Well, if you're willing to try, so am I," I said excitedly.

It seemed fated to be when a few days later, Zachary and Joe both mentioned wanting a little brother for Christmas. Well, I hadn't let them down on Zachary's Christmas wish for a dad—hopefully we could grant them this wish too.

Soon after our talk we started trying to conceive in earnest. Tanya and I always had a fulfilling physical relationship. Thanks to Sally's friendship and guidance so many years ago, I knew I could have a satisfying sexual relationship. Now our marital fun together had a special purpose. We tried for about six months with no result, so in May we scheduled an appointment with my doctor to discuss it.

The doctor told us, "Tanya should try and have this baby before she turns 35," which was only 15 months away. He explained the best days for trying based on

Tanya's cycle, then wrote me a prescription for a stronger dosage of Viagra—I already took a lower dosage, but as the doctor handed us the new prescription he said smiling, "Let's get 'er done!" His terminology may have been unorthodox, but I hoped he was right. We kept trying.

Late that June, my family got some horrible news. My cousin Steve's oldest son, Fred, had been killed in a car accident. He and his wife were expecting a baby that summer, and we were all crushed. The funeral was planned for the afternoon of Thursday, July 1.

That Saturday, the whole family would gather at my house on Kerr Lake for our annual Fourth of July barbecue. Our annual tradition was to hold a pig-picking barbecue. We roasted a whole split pig on an outdoor grill, which made the meat so tender that everyone could pick out the bits they liked best. This year it would take on special significance because we would be together to celebrate Fred's life and comfort each other.

It was the end of the second quarter at the bank and I had a lot of work to complete, so I stayed at home that day to focus. This would make it easier for Tanya and me to travel to Fred's funeral in the afternoon. As I sat in my home office, typing away at the computer, Tanya came in and set something on the keyboard with a little click.

I didn't even look up, figuring she had just come in to return a pencil. When I realized she was still in the room, I tore my eyes from the screen and looked at her. She was grinning sheepishly.

"What do you need?"

— ⚡ —

She just smiled and gestured toward the keyboard. I looked down and saw it wasn't a pencil she'd put down, but a pregnancy test. It took me a few moments to realize what the blue plus-sign meant.

I couldn't believe it. "You're lying. You're not pregnant," I finally managed to say.

She kept on smiling.

My head was spinning and my heart felt ready to burst with joy. Could I truly be getting yet another blessing in my already full life? "Wow. Oh, wow! We've got to tell everyone!"

"No, Bryant, we can't tell anyone until I make sure. Sometimes these things aren't accurate. I've scheduled a doctor's appointment today after the funeral, so don't say a word till then."

I sighed. "This is going to be hard."

"I'm pretty sure I am pregnant though," she said. "I've been feeling so tired lately, and kind of nauseated."

I knew it was smart to wait until she had seen the doctor, and the focus of the day was remembering Fred, so I kept my mouth shut.

When Tanya got home from her doctor's appointment, she was smiling again. "I'm definitely pregnant!" she said.

It felt like fireworks going off inside my head, I was so excited. Late that afternoon, I saw my parents in the yard and hollered for them to come over for a minute.

"So, Mom, what do you think about being a grandma?" I asked casually.

"Well, I like it," she said.

I gave her a look and she continued in confusion. "I *am* a grandma. What are you talking about?" I started to grin and watched her expression change as my words sank in. "Wait, you're kidding. You can't be serious. Is Tanya…?" By this point, both of us were smiling.

"Well, congratulations! I think?" Mom said. "You have a lot going on in your lives. Can you handle this okay?" We reassured her that yes, we could—we'd discussed it and knew we'd need some extra help from both sets of parents, as well as from the twins, but we wanted a baby together.

Dad had no second thoughts. "I want a girl. After the first year, she's all mine!" Many of the children in both Tanya's family and mine are boys.

"Please don't tell anyone else," I said. "Tanya and I want to make an announcement about it on Saturday at the barbecue. Hopefully it will help raise everyone's spirits. So just keep it a secret."

After they left, I called Thom and asked him to come over. Upon his arrival, I handed him a cigar and asked, "You ready to be grandpa again?"

He looked a bit startled. "You're kidding, right?"

His look implied that I must be nuts. I realized he was genuinely concerned that us having a baby was unwise. After raising his own two children then helping with the twins for several years, he seemed ready to be done with babies. I realized he probably wished we'd talked with him about our decision. That he could have had reservations never occurred to me.

As we talked further, he said, "I can see how excited you are, man. I have my concerns, but I really am happy for you both."

"I understand where you're coming from, and I'm sorry we didn't say anything about our plans sooner. We were both surprised by Tanya's test though—we weren't sure it would happen and just found out today. We're going to tell everyone on Saturday at the lake."

We arrived at the lake on Friday to prepare the food for the next day. I did let the news slip to John and Anne that afternoon but I knew I could trust them. I also called my cousin Lynda. She was an important presence in my life. She'd been my playmate as a child and after my injury had led some of the efforts to fundraise for my family's medical expenses. We'd worked together for nearly twenty years. She was more than a cousin—she was a dear friend. I knew she couldn't come to the barbecue, so I wanted her to hear the news from me first. I called under the pretense of checking on the second quarter report's progress.

"Lynda, is everything okay at the office?" I asked

"Yes sir," she replied cheerfully. "Is something up?"

"I've got some good news for you. Tanya and I are—" was all I managed to say before she started going crazy, shrieking in excitement on the other end of the line.

"You're lying!" she finally shouted before bursting into tears of joy.

Lynda had always known my dream of wanting a child and had been asking me whether we were going to have a baby since we'd gotten married—yet the news still reduced her to a blubbering mess.

"You have to promise to keep this a secret," I told her. "We're telling everyone else at the barbecue tomorrow, and I'll tell the folks at the office on Monday."

The mood at the barbecue was somber, but being together seemed to help everyone cope. Tanya and I planned to make a little announcement about the baby once most of the relatives arrived. My parents had done a great job of keeping it a secret until Dad's sister Betty came and put her hand on Tanya's shoulder. Tanya looked up and saw her smiling with tears in her eyes.

"Uh oh," said Tanya. "You know, don't you? Who told you?"

"Jimmy told me and Glenice," she said.

Tanya motioned me over. "Bryant, Glenice and Betty know. Your dad let it slip. You have to tell your family, quick, before your dad spills the beans to everyone else."

I looked over at Dad, who quickly busied himself cooking the hush puppies, and shook my head with a smile. "Aunt Betty, don't you or Glenice say a word,"

"You better tell everyone soon, or else our kids will be mad that we found out before they did," said Aunt Betty. "Congratulations, by the way!"

A few minutes later, I had managed to round everyone up. "Everyone, can I have your attention?"

Everyone quieted down.

"This week has been hell for the Neville clan. On Thursday, we laid to rest Fred, a young man just starting his adult life with his new wife who is soon having their first child. None of us can know why this happened, but someday, we will find meaning in this tragedy."

I swallowed a lump in my throat and went on.

"Fred helped Dad build my house, and he and I had an opportunity one afternoon to talk about death and how we'd like to be remembered. I'm sure he hadn't intended that conversation be relevant so soon, but he told me he hoped folks wouldn't just sit around sadly. He wanted a party with stories about the fun times. So today is for Fred—no tears of sadness allowed."

Many of my family members were smiling. I pressed on.

"Now, to start things off on the right foot, I want to call to mind the wise saying that when one door closes, another opens. No one can ever take Fred's place, but in about eight months, Tanya and I will be bringing the newest member of our family into the world!"

Jaws dropped. Several people gasped. A few started to cry happy tears. My news caught everyone off guard, and Tanya and I found ourselves bombarded with congratulatory hugs, handshakes, and pats on the back. The news had put a positive glow on the day and made everyone's hearts a little lighter. We wouldn't find out the baby's sex for a few months, but already many were betting on a girl.

As we shared the news of Tanya's pregnancy with friends, quite a few people were surprised, and I'm sure many wondered if we'd used a medical procedure to facilitate the process. Just like me at age 17, many people have no idea that individuals with a spinal cord injury often can still have sex. I hoped that seeing my full, well-rounded life would help change the common misconception that a spinal cord injury or similar disability is akin to a sentence of life imprisonment in a broken body.

Tanya's first pregnancy with the boys had been easy, but now she was having problems. In August, she was constantly nauseated and dehydrated. It wasn't just morning sickness—she vomited several times a day and couldn't keep any food down. The doctor tried several different medications that didn't help, and after a week she ended up in the hospital because of dehydration.

This was a rough period. For the first time, Tanya and I argued.

Finally the doctor put a peripherally inserted central catheter, called a PICC line, into her right bicep so she could intravenously receive the nutrients and electrolytes she needed from a bag of solution. It was like a permanent IV that she carried around with her in a backpack. During this time she often worked from home, so she could rest during the day if needed.

This was a rough period and the first time in our marriage that Tanya and I argued. Even though the PICC line was giving Tanya and the baby all the nutrients they needed, I'd still try to coax her to eat a little something. I remembered my own days right after the accident in the ICU when I was NPO and how excited I was to finally have a proper meal. I imagined she must feel the same way.

"You need to eat. Why don't you try to have a little something?"

She shot me a look. "What's the point? I'm just going to throw it up anyway."

"Maybe, but don't you think you ought to try and eat something?"

"Bryant, I'm getting the nutrients I need from the IV. Eating something will make me feel worse. Please! Just leave me alone!"

Emotions ran high and there were some tears, but by late October she felt much better, had the PICC line removed, and returned to the office.

During one of her October doctor's appointments, we had an ultrasound to learn the baby's sex. Tanya's family traditionally liked being surprised, but Tanya realized I would drive her nuts if we didn't know.

Everyone was convinced that this high-maintenance pregnancy meant it was a girl, but the night before the appointment I reconsidered. In horse racing, conventional wisdom dictates that when everyone bets on one horse, you should go the opposite way. I decided to switch my vote and bet on a boy.

My instincts were right! It was so exciting to look at the screen and see my son. During the first few ultrasounds, he had looked like a little peanut, but now we could see his head, arms, and legs. It was remarkable to think that in just a few months, he'd be here with us. Zachary and Joe were excited too—they figured a little brother would be more interested in sports than a little sister.

We planned to name him Kenneth Dale. Kenneth was Tanya's Uncle Jeff's middle name, and Dale was after Dale Earnhardt, Sr. Both of these men had been important and inspirational to the two of us, so we wanted to honor their legacies with our son's name. If we had had a girl, her name would have been Kathleen Rose, after Great-Aunt Steen and Tanya's Grandmother Rose.

During this time, we relied on our parents for help with our daily routine. We anticipated needing help in Tanya's third trimester, but her illness made it virtually impossible for her to do much of anything only three months into the pregnancy.

Thom had always come over to help Tanya get me

out of bed and dressed. The fact that I'm 6'4" and weigh about 250 pounds made it challenging. Tanya could do this alone normally, but it was easier with a second set of hands. They used a mesh sling, almost like a seat, connected by chains to a moveable lift that was cranked to raise me from the bed then lower me into the wheelchair. Now Thom came over and helped me into bed at night as well.

I also needed to be rolled over in the middle of the night. I sleep on my side, with a pillow between my knees and sheepskin booties that prevent my feet from rubbing together. All this helps prevent pressure sores. After four hours asleep on one side, Tanya would roll me over onto my other side to redistribute my weight. Now our fathers took turns coming over around 2 o'clock in the morning to make sure I was rolled over.

This was a huge imposition on both of them—even more so on Thom because he was younger and helped with this task more often than my father. I knew Thom was apprehensive about the pregnancy and hated having to ask him to do more to help us, but he gladly pitched in. My mother had once again taken over my catheter and bowel program regimens. I was incredibly grateful to my parents and in-laws for their help.

Over the years, my parents had worked hard and made many sacrifices to help me live a productive, happy life, and never once complained. I knew certain tasks were harder for my parents as they got older, so I tried to help when I could. I hired someone to mow my parents' lawn and pitched in with other expenses.

I never outgrew my love of giving surprise gifts, so I treated them to things whenever I could. I surprised

Dad with a new pickup truck, which brought tears to his eyes—one of the only times I can remember seeing him cry. Mom loved Tim McGraw, so when a local radio station ran a Christmas wish contest, I wrote to them about how she'd cared for me all my life and wanted to attend Tim's concert. Not only did Mom get front-row seats, she also got to meet him before the show. I was sure that having a biological grandchild they could play with and love from day one was the greatest gift I could give them.

Sometimes Tanya worried about how she would take care of me after the baby was born, but our parents promised they'd be there to help whenever needed and the boys promised to help too. My biggest worry was how I'd afford to feed three boys—the twins already seemed to eat as much as ten children.

Before Kenneth was born, we decided to build a third bedroom for Joe to move into, so we could use his room for Kenneth. I designed and Dad built this room inside the attached two-car garage. It connected to the rest of the house through a hallway in the kitchen. When Joe saw how naturally the room fit into the home's layout, he got excited to move.

The room was finished in mid-February, and not a moment too soon. Tanya's official due date was March 7, but between the trouble she'd had with her pregnancy and her previous delivery by Cesarean, the doctors scheduled a Cesarean delivery for Kenneth, to prevent labor complications. They chose February 24—by then, he'd be fully grown. This sounded like a fine date to me, since 24 was my lucky number. My birthday was October 24, my wedding anniversary was May 24, and now my son would be born February 24.

This made life easier for us. Since we now knew when to expect the big day, we could adjust my care routine accordingly. If Tanya had unexpectedly gone into labor, we might have been left scrambling.

The night of February 23, my neighbors from Kerr Lake, John and Anne, arrived. We had to arrive at Southside Regional Medical Center at 5:15 in the morning, which was about a half hour away, so we started our routine at 3 o'clock. Tanya showered and dressed, Thom and John helped me get out of bed and ready, and then Juanita came to stay with the boys while we went to the hospital in the van. My mother drove separately and met us there.

Suddenly Tanya's blood pressure dropped and her skin paled. The baby's heartbeat dropped too. I was terrified.

After we checked in, they sat Tanya in a wheelchair and we went upstairs to her room. The night shift crew was still working, and one of the night nurses said, "I'll let the five of you go back for now, but once it gets busier, there can only be two of you in the room."

The nurses put Tanya in bed and started prepping her. Her blood pressure dropped, so she had to lie back for a few minutes until it stabilized and they could continue their work. They were having some trouble putting in her IV when suddenly her blood pressure dropped very low and her skin paled. The baby's heartbeat dropped too. I was terrified.

The room quickly filled with people, and my fears

subsided when the doctor administered a medication that raised Tanya's blood pressure. After a few minutes she and the baby were okay. When the day shift nurses came on, my family and I found that we knew quite a few of them, so the rules about guests went out the window.

Around 8:30 that morning, they wheeled Tanya across the hall to the delivery room. One of the nurses wrapped me, chair and all, in a hospital gown, then put a surgical cap and mask on me. I waited in the hall while the nurses gave Tanya a spinal block, then one of them came out and said, "We're ready for you." My heart was pounding in excitement. This was it!

I went into the room with a vision of how deliveries look on TV and in movies, where the husband sits by his wife's side holding her hand, looking down toward her feet. This was nothing like a movie—when I rolled in, there was no room for me by Tanya's bedside and the doctor was about to make the incision across her belly, so I parked my chair at the foot of the bed. I had a clear view of the instrument table and everything Dr. Roberts was doing, but I couldn't see Tanya's face, as a small curtain across her midsection blocked her from my view.

"You're not squeamish, are you?" Dr. Roberts asked as he started cutting. I didn't think so, but I certainly never imagined I'd be watching a doctor cutting into my wife. The incision didn't bleed much, and I sighed in relief. This wasn't so bad.

Then he cut across Tanya's uterus. I've never seen so much blood in my life, and I was once again horrified. There was no way anyone could survive so much bleeding, but no one else seemed worried so I quickly calmed down. The nurses suctioned up the blood, and

one of them said, "Okay, you're about to see your baby!"
Dr. Roberts reached down and pulled out my son,
holding him tightly by the back and throat.

My God! This doctor was going to choke my son to
death! But babies are tougher than I thought, because
they suctioned out his mouth and I heard a mighty cry.

"He's perfect!" one of the nurses said.

A wave of emotions, building for nine months,
finally washed over me. Tears filled my eyes as the nurse
wrapped him in a blanket and placed him on my tray,
still covered in blood and crying his heart out. His eyes
were still closed, and as he paused to take a breath, he
stretched out his arms and rested his tiny hand on my

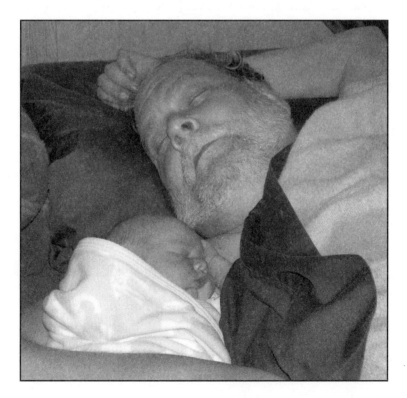

beard.

For a few seconds, the world stood still. Thirty years ago, one doctor told me my life was over. Now another doctor had just handed me my life's greatest dream. I thanked God for giving me this perfect baby boy.

I smiled at my son. "Hello, Kenneth," I whispered.

The nurses cleaned Kenneth and let Tanya hold him for a few minutes, then I left the room. Tanya and I didn't want her to chance going through another difficult pregnancy, so the doctor was going to tie her tubes.

As I rolled into the hallway, I could see my mother peeking out of Tanya's room. The room was packed with my family—aunts, cousins, everyone patiently waiting for Kenneth to make his debut. When the nurse finally brought him over, she let me hold him while everyone gathered around to meet him. After ten minutes they took him to the nursery to be weighed and examined and get some shots.

The next few days flew by. The boys went to visit their mother and meet their new brother, and other relatives dropped by too. Tanya and Kenneth came home on Sunday and we all began to adjust to our new family member.

The second night he was home, Kenneth was restless. Tanya was exhausted and brought him into the bedroom, where I was already lying in bed. She snuggled him against my chest and wrapped my arm securely around him. He calmed down and finally fell asleep. I didn't sleep much. I just lay there, watching my beautiful baby sleep and feeling like I was in a dream.

Zachary and Joe were excited to be big brothers.

They adored Kenneth from the moment they met him and loved caring for him, carrying him around the house and feeding him his bottle. They quickly learned that helping with Kenneth meant they could get out of other chores—"I've got the baby, Joe, so you need to empty the dishwasher." Clever boys!

Kenneth loved the attention, smiling constantly. I

Despite my paralysis, we found creative ways for me to help care for Kenneth. When he was an infant, I was able to hold him on a pillow on my wheelchair tray, with a bottle of formula held against my chin.

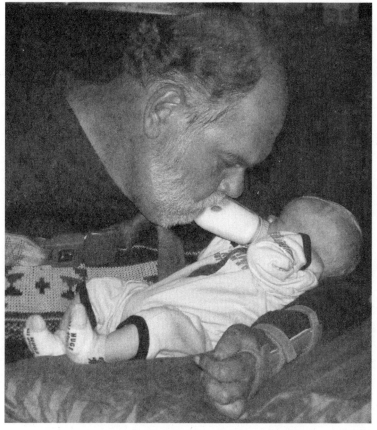

never saw a happier baby. My hearted melted every time he looked at me with his big deep-blue eyes and smiled.

There were some rough moments too—sleepless nights, crying spells, frazzled nerves. We were often exhausted and sometimes Tanya felt overwhelmed, but I was an expert at patience and knew that now my son's needs often had to come first. I'd spent many years doubting I'd ever get to have the fatherhood experience, so I thought every moment of it was wonderful.

On April 17, we baptized Kenneth. We had originally planned it for April 24—I was tickled at having yet another 24 in my lineup of meaningful dates—but that was Easter Sunday, which would have made for a hectic day between the baptism and our usual church services, so we held it a week earlier. Now all three of my sons had been baptized into Bott Memorial Presbyterian Church. I was committed to leading the boys in a meaningful and moral life.

I enjoyed watching each of Kenneth's milestones: sitting up, standing up, starting to crawl, and especially his first words: "mama" and "dada." When he was a newborn, someone would put a pillow on my tray so he could nap with me in my chair. When he got too big for naps on my tray, someone would stand him on it, holding his hands for balance, and he and I would have a nice long conversation at least once a day.

After six weeks, Tanya returned to work. Juanita kept Kenneth during the day and stayed with the boys whenever school was out. My mother came over a lot too—she just couldn't get enough of Kenneth, saying he looked just like me when I was a baby. Now when she arrived at our house, she gave me a quick greeting and went right to the baby. Dad couldn't wait for Kenneth to get bigger so they could play catch.

I hope to pass on to my boys a few lessons that have helped me stay positive and undefeated.

Now that Kenneth had arrived, I wanted to complete the adoption process for Zachary and Joe and officially make them my sons. William D. Allen, III, an attorney who is the chairman of the bank's board, offered to help me fill out the legal paperwork and guide me through the process. He knew the judge handling the case and offered to meet with him personally about it.

Thanks to the character reference Mr. Allen provided, I was spared the lengthy background check, and in May of 2011, I officially became the boys' father. The twins had always felt like my sons, but now they were mine in the eyes of the law. My family truly was complete now.

My parents are my role models for how to raise my sons, and they continue to inspire me to be the best father possible. They never gave up on me and were just as determined as I was to prove that callous doctor wrong. Every day I thank God for blessing me with such loving and dedicated parents.

Mom and Dad taught me to be kind to others, use common sense, be honest, and think for myself. Their only expectation for me was having a happy life, and that's the same thing I want for Joseph, Zachary, and Kenneth. Just like my parents, my priority is spending time with my boys and being involved in their lives. I aspire to give them a house full of love just like I had growing up.

I hope to pass on to my boys a few important life lessons that have helped me stay positive and undefeated, even in my darkest moments. A situation can be either an obstacle or an opportunity, depending on how you react. Work hard, even if it's uncomfortable or unpleasant, and don't give up on yourself or your dreams. Never judge a person based on their appearance, for it can be deceiving. And finally, learn to laugh at yourself and don't take things too seriously.

My life changed in the blink of an eye one chilly night 30 years ago, but thanks to the love and support of my family and friends, my faith, and my determination, my spinal cord injury never defined or defeated me.

Instead of seeing the world as full of limitations, I see it as full of possibilities. I may have achieved my dreams rolling on four wheels instead of walking on two legs, but I wouldn't trade my journey for anything.

epilogue

Throughout our lives we each face numerous challenges. Some are overcome easily, while others take much longer to struggle through and have long-term consequences. Then there are those that alter the course of an individual's life: an accident, a serious illness, or some other trauma.

How you deal with these life-changing circumstances is ultimately up to you. How you feel about yourself sets the stage for how your family and friends will react: if you refuse to give up on yourself, others will follow your lead. The greatest leaders in the world acknowledge that the key to success is surrounding themselves with people they trust and treating these individuals well to ensure they stay. Regardless of your challenge, remain positive, do not shut out those around you, and never give up on your hopes and dreams—no matter how impossible they may seem. And most importantly, never forget how to laugh at yourself. Sometimes laughter is the best and only medicine available.

My purpose in writing this book is to help others understand that their lives don't have to end in the face of such life-altering challenges. My experience has been with a spinal cord injury, but the lessons I learned hold true for the majority of disabilities, illnesses, and other difficulties. The mission of the National Spinal Cord Injury Association (NSCIA), the outreach arm of the United Spinal Association, is virtually the same: to enable people with spinal cord injuries or disorders to achieve their highest level of independence, health, and personal fulfillment. Because we share such a similar goal, NSCIA and I have partnered to use my story in inspiring others to never give up on themselves and their dreams. I am humbled to be their partner in spreading this important message.

A good person did me a very nice deed several years ago and explained I could pay him back by one day helping another in need. If I have touched a few lives with these pages, I hope, in part, to have satisfied that debt.

resources

These organizations and websites can assist those affected by spinal cord injury and other disabilities. They also provide information for caretakers and the general public.

UNITED SPINAL ASSOCIATION'S mission is to improve the quality of life of all people living with spinal cord injuries and disorders (SCI/D). Today, United Spinal is the largest non-profit organization dedicated to helping people living with SCI/D. It is committed to providing active-lifestyle information, peer support, and advocacy that empower individuals to achieve their highest potential in all facets of life. Phone: 718-803-3782 Email: info@unitedspinal.org Website: unitedspinal.org

Other United Spinal Association programs include:

NATIONAL SPINAL CORD INJURY ASSOCIATION'S mission is to improve the quality of life of all people living with spinal cord injuries and disorders (SCI/D). It is the membership division of United Spinal Association. NSCIA is the portal through which individuals and organizations can be involved in the organization. NSCIA connects people living with SCI/D across the country. Countless members benefit from the experience of others who have lived through similar challenges—and many remain involved to share their knowledge and experience with people new to the community. Phone: 718-803-3782 Website: www.spinalcord.org info@unitedspinal.org

VETSFIRST directly assists veterans and their eligible family members in obtaining the benefits they are entitled to, deserve, and need. VetsFirst's network of National Service Officers provides free assistance, resources, and representation for veterans struggling to navigate the intricate and often confusing VA claims process. In addition to providing individual support and counseling services, VetsFirst offers timely news and information across the spectrum of issues presently impacting veterans, including guides on self-help, state benefits, separating from the military, and exclusive feature stories on military health care and VA funding and compensation. (718) 803-3782, vetsfirst.org

USERSFIRST advocates for greater access to appropriate wheelchairs, mobility scooters, and seating systems for people with disabilities. UsersFirst rejects the one-size-fits-all perception of mobility equipment and believes that the right wheelchairs, mobility scooters, and seating systems are fundamental elements in maintaining the health, quality of life, and independence of people with disabilities. The UsersFirst Movement gains momentum through United Spinal Association's wide-range of programs and services; public policy initiatives; large peer support network and growing list of national chapters; highly visible web presence; and lifestyle and educational publications that reach hundreds of thousands of individuals with disabilities annually. (718) 803-3782, Website: usersfirst.org

ABLE TO TRAVEL provides knowledgeable travel agents that have dealt with all types of issues that a traveler using a wheelchair or who has limited mobility may encounter during a trip. (888) 211-3635 Website: abletotravel.org

NEW MOBILITY is the magazine for active wheelchair users. It encourages the integration of active-lifestyle wheelchair users into mainstream society, while simultaneously reflecting the vibrant world of disability-related arts, media, advocacy, and philosophy. (888) 850-0344 ext. 209 newmobility.com

WHEELCHAIR MEDIC offers both sales and service for all wheelchairs and mobility scooters. It is one of the largest wheelchair and mobility equipment repair companies in the nation. They also offer a full line of lift chairs, walkers, portable ramps, shower chairs, tub benches, handheld shower heads, and many other devices that enhance activities of daily living. (718) 352-1623 Email: info@wheelchairmedic.com, wheelchairmedic.com

USA TECHGUIDE is a webguide to wheelchairs, mobility scooters, and assistive technology choices. You can read and submit wheelchair reviews, mobility scooter reviews, wheelchair cushion reviews, standing device reviews, and search The TechGuide for all types of assistive equipment., www.usatechguide.org

ACCESSIBILITY SERVICES provides consulting services devoted exclusively to making the built environment accessible to people with disabilities. Their team of professional accessibility consultants conduct plan reviews, site assessments, and training that get any project through the myriad of state and federal accessibility requirements to successful completion. (718) 803-3782 ext. 7502 info@accessibility-services.com, accessibility-services.com